**SPORT**

Physical Th
Instructional ......

# THE FLEXIBILITY MANUAL

by Jean M. Peters, B.S., P.T.
Howard K. Peters, Jr. B.S., P.T.

*Life begins with mobility and
ends with immobility.
In between lies the quality of one's life.*

Sports Kinetics, Inc.

725 Hillside Ave.

Berwyn, PA 19312-1702

(610) 647-3299

Library of Congress Cataloging-in-Publication Data

Jean M. Peters, BS, PT, and Howard K. Peters, Jr., BS, PT

THE FLEXIBILITY MANUAL, 2nd Edition
1. Flexibility.
2. Mobility.
3. Reciprocal Innervation.
4. Inhibition.
5. Physical Therapy.
6. Sports Conditioning.
7. Exercise

ISBN: 0-9633896-0-2

Don't pick up THE FLEXIBILITY MANUAL hoping to find "secrets" for addressing specific injuries. It was designed to impress on you the importance of physical mobility and to show you how to regain and maintain it in a sensible manner. Don't put it down without understanding these benefits. You will be well rewarded.

# CONTENTS

# ABOUT THE AUTHORS

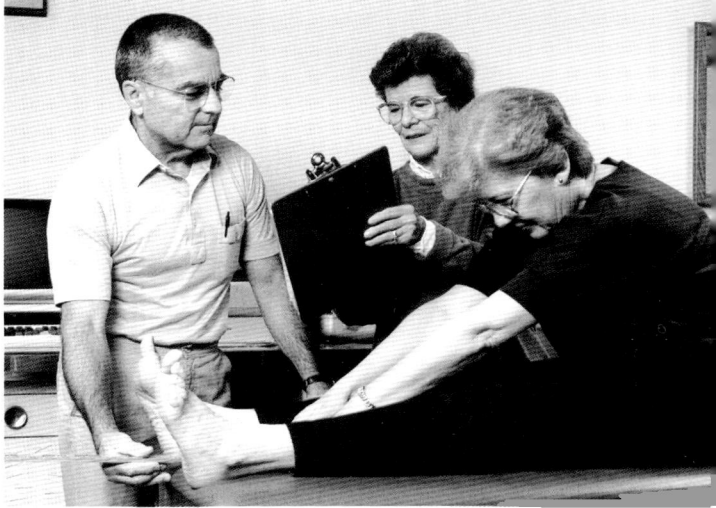

Jean and Pete Peters are a Physical Therapy team. Their experience with neuromuscular disabilities has been gained from epidemic polio treatment, children and adults with brain damage, general orthopedics, and sports-medicine.

Personal and family interest in individual and team sports, treatment of athletic injuries, and applications of accumulated experience with the neuromuscular system has led them to establish their SPORTS KINETICS Health and Sports Science facility. Here they not only provide evaluation and rehabilitation of athletic injuries, but uniquely extend a service of education and preventive medicine for nonathletes as well as athletes.

# PREFACE

What is SPORTS KINETICS? It is a progressive concept of health and sports science undergoing constant change. One aspect is its re-examination of existing approaches to health and sports conditioning. Another aspect is its continual development of scientific methods for fitness and human performance. Most importantly, it represents the application of these concepts. All programs undergo continual development and change according to the needs of the active and not-so-active members of the community.

Lectures and demonstrations on the care and prevention of injuries are conducted for coaches and athletes. Entire sports teams, e.g., basketball, hockey, lacrosse, gymnastics, soccer, football, volleyball, etc. are physically profiled. Physical profiles for runners, cyclists, swimmers, scullers, and other individual sports people enable them, also, to assess their training procedures with measurable performance data. The aim is not to teach skills, but to make athletes more physically aware and fit individuals for benefit of themselves and their coaches.

Health and sports science are compatible, non-discriminatory, and of benefit to athlete and nonathlete alike. It is the goal of Sports Kinetics to convey this concept to everyone.

During the planning stages of our facility, we were taken aback to realize how ill-founded the existing methods of stretching were. The best assumptions were, and still are, inadequate approaches. They fail on all counts and by no means could they be accepted for a program of prevention. We had to devise an original and complete method – something basic, simple, safe.

In our estimation, consideration of the physiological action of muscle fibers has been much too casual. We do not mean the detailed clinical examination and laboratory kinesiology, but the function of muscles when related to actual sports movements. It is disturbing to see the incomplete preparations taken by individuals to pursue their sports and the manner in which stretching is conducted on amateur and professional levels. It easily can be a disaster for an eager reader to apply most of the stretching methods presented in the current literature.

This book was developed from our Sports Kinetics fitness and athletic performance programs. Such a presentation does not assure that we know it all. To the contrary, we have analyzed and reapplied the method to so many athletes and nonathletes that we know that we do not know everything. Our work is not finished, but at this stage explaining the success of our method should evoke interest, and we hope it will inspire further refinements in flexibility training.

# INTRODUCTION

Flexibility is what we all had as children, and we must be envious as we watch a small child in his or her activities – reminders of our lost mobility. At Sports Kinetics, we prefer conditioning our athletes at 11 years of age or older. We believe that flexibility considerations should include even pre-schoolers. Many children at six years of age already present limited extensibility of their hamstring muscles. We attribute this to a primary role of these muscles in running – conceivably the first sports activity of every child. It would be nice to see flexibility training a major part of the physical education classes offered to our school students. At least at age six years and older it could counteract the undesirable effects of their sitting at desks and make them aware of the value of maintaining mobility throughout their lives.

One small private school of approximately 215 students K-12 has followed our program since 1984. We, within our lifetimes, don't anticipate substantiating the benefits to them in their later years. We only can observe the mobility safely regained and maintained by all ages of participants. The male and female members of its ten varsity sports teams have suffered no muscle strain (non-contact) injuries.

Looking at a broad spectrum of physical growth and development from the vantage point of our fitness and athletic performance programs, the authors recognize additional serious loss of flexibility as a result of the growth spurt of late childhood. The length of the muscles and elasticity of the joint connective tissues do not automatically keep pace with bone growth. In some unusual cases, the disparity has been devastating from the aspect of sports participation.

The greatest incidence of playing time loss throughout all age groups of athletes is due to minor, and not so minor, injuries related to the lack of flexibility. The disappointment of missing competition lingers well beyond the recovery time of a disabling muscle strain.

Following the termination of organized sports in high school or college, as our sports-minded individuals enter the work force, there is an abrupt decrease in exercise opportunity, and sports participation is delayed for many reasons. Many individuals recognize their loss of physical conditioning but resist the call to fitness. A toll is taken by the sedentary position behind the desk or wheel of a car or in front of the TV. Sporadic or weekend sports do not promote fitness or prevent injuries, and in this category some of our more irreversible abuses occur as our bodies seem to become increasingly less forgiving and reparative.

As the age of retirement approaches, we become conditioned (mentally, that is) to accept further slowing of our activities – athletic and otherwise. Yet we see contradictions to this – notably Masters and Seniors programs. Many who train for and participate in these events are athletes who never stopped in their attempts to maintain fitness. Others have regained it. Obviously, loss of mobility is *not* a normal process of aging and premature slowing to a halt is not necessarily our fate. A fuller life is a proven possibility. However, a commitment is required.

So, this has been our goal in developing our Sports Kinetics flexibility training method: to present a reasoned exercise format, based upon research and clinical observation, which will be applicable to any of the aforementioned stages of inflexibility.

The authors wish to thank not only those contributors who actually helped to produce this manual, but the many known and unknown athletes and individuals who have inspired us to consider their needs.

We can not consider this work to be the final word in flexibillity training, but will continue to examine theory and practice to serve a more physically active society and its evermore demanding athletes.

Having put a great deal of effort into this book, we ask you to accept our application of terminology which might differ from that of other authors. Some definitions might appear to be merely a matter of semantics. However, they have provided a working format for us in our programs, and we feel comfortable with them. Other terminology might be considered new and will have to earn acceptance.

# STRETCHING IN SPORTS

Athletes are not the only ones whose performance suffers from inflexibility. It is reflected in all age groups and obviously increases the longer it is ignored. The result is loss of mobility and function.

The authors criticize existing presentations of flexibility as a means of reducing sports injuries. Most serious works cover physiology adequately. It is the lack of consideration of physiological principles which elicits the criticism. So many athletes and individuals are admonished to stretch, but the application of the methods and the methods themselves are at fault. There are still too many injuries, at all levels of sports, resulting from flexibility training as presently applied.

As you become acquainted with "active" stretching, you will begin to look at current applications of stretching with increasing skepticism. Utilizing our human nervous system which has evolved over eons, rather than ignoring and defiantly opposing it, will make sense. You will question more of the features of present-day stretching and recognize some other problems.

For example, two exercises for which we have no enthusiasm are the "hurdler's stretch" and "hanging ten." We mention them only because they are recommended so frequently. You also may notice some other contradictions in the following photographs.

The anterior and posterior cruciate ligaments serve to stabilize the knee joint when it is extended. We do not like the unnecessary forces placed upon the other ligaments and structures of the knee joint when it is flexed and the lower leg is rotated externally as in the hurdler's stretch in the photograph below.

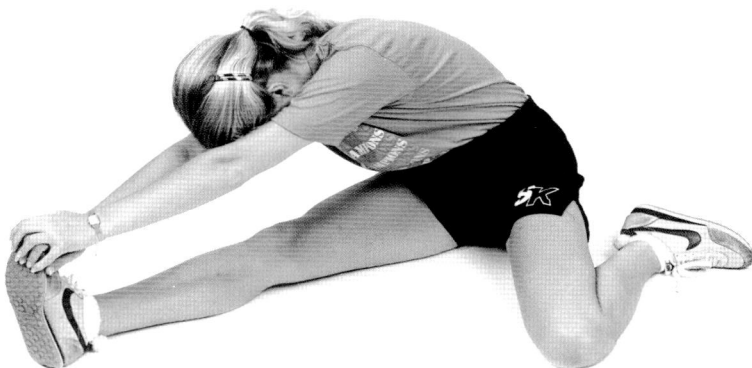

Hanging ten toes on the edge of a step is not so effective a stretch as it seems. The weight of the body on the heel cords requires controlling contractions by the lower leg muscles thereby depreciating the intended benefits.

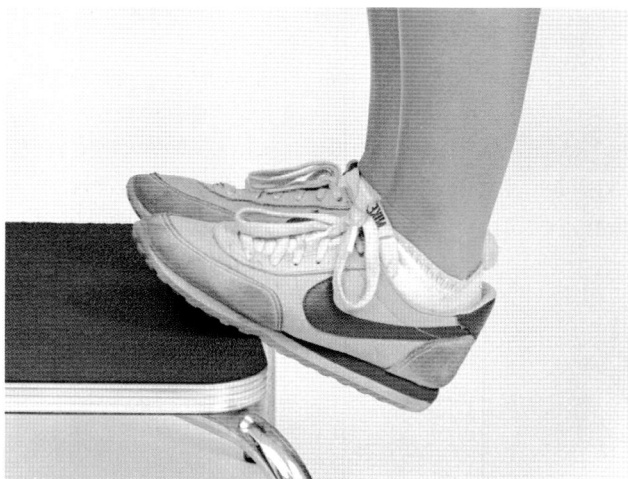

It should not have to be said that the quick fix is seldom that at all.

While working your way through our entire program, you undoubtedly will notice similarities to many of the stretching positions currently in use. It is the application of the exercises which is so significantly different.

As you read about and apply our "active" methods, you will understand our objections to your or anyone else's pulling on your muscles to stretch them.

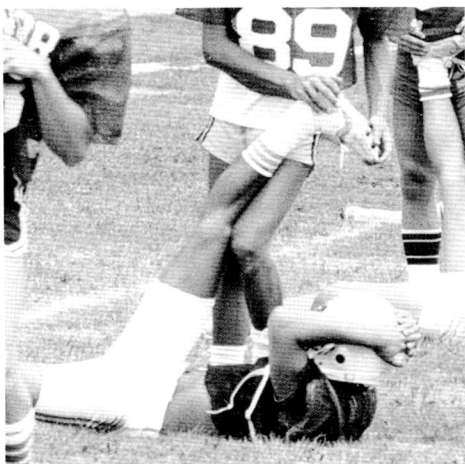

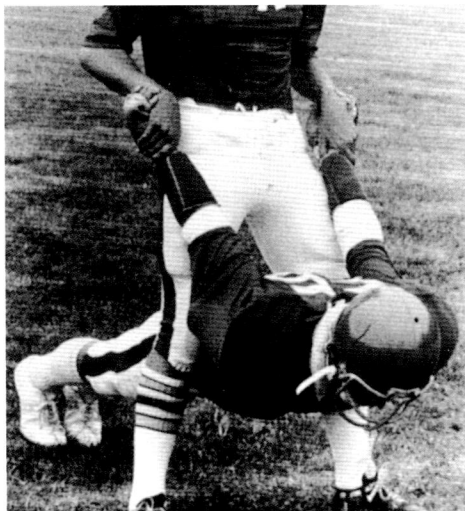

Flexibility exercises cannot be considered normal functional positions of daily activities. So, naturally, reasonable care must be taken. An exercise either is performed comfortably or is deferred until it can be done so. Each exercise of a group is in progressive sequence, and the preceding one helps in achieving the next.

Our declaration is that flexibility is one of the most important factors in the prevention of athletic injuries. Of course, you don't have to be an athlete to suffer the consequences of immobility. The athlete's awareness usually comes suddenly, the result of an injury, while the nonathlete's problem is insidious, culminating over a longer period of neglect. Without mobility, *the most important component of fitness*, the other systems of the body cannot be improved or maintained satisfactorily. The human body, utilized for sports or work activities, should be maintained at its optimal level of full ranges of joint motion. Otherwise, stress forces – either as anticipated and intentional muscle contractions or as unguarded and accidental movements – could be excessive. Such injury can involve supportive rotary mechanisms (joint connective tissues) and more linear type mechanisms (muscles and tendons). Even minimal forces applied to musculoskeletal structures with limited range of motion can cause damage when the impetus cannot be spent (decelerated) through a full range.

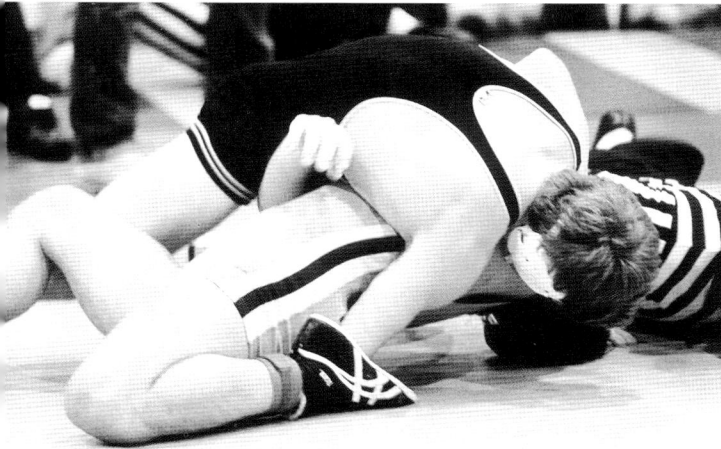

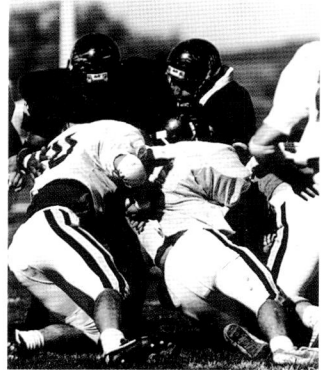

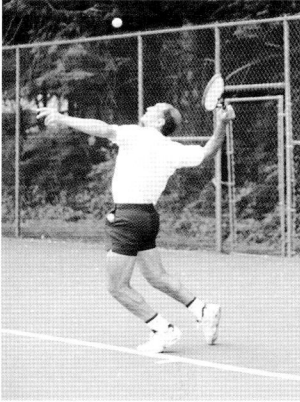

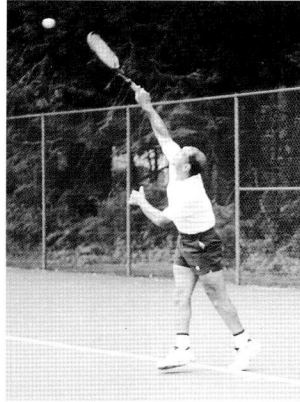

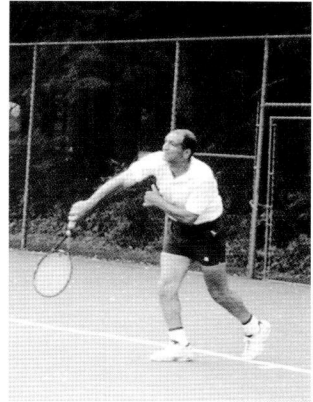

Some forces, accepted as part of the sports environment, can be absorbed without the athlete's sustaining injury, but others are excessive and cause injury, which is classed as accidental. The goal, then, is to avoid the avoidable and reduce the incidence of "accidental" injuries.

It must be emphasized that neither muscle strength nor flexibility is the panacea for prevention of athletic injuries, but flexibility presently is the most neglected area of athletic fitness and begs for attention. The number of proponents of stretching for flexibility as a safety measure in sports is increasing. The consensus appears to be that it's important and should be practiced by more athletes and nonathletes alike. However, what has been missing in such pronouncements is a rational application of what, how, when, and why. What some proponents consider necessary for one sport may not apply fully to another sport if flexibility is approached from such a singular viewpoint. Would not achievement of total body flexibility be a wiser approach? Then, when a specific sport or incident tends to limit mobility in certain muscles and joint structures, it will be recognized, and the individual can concentrate more on those areas. For example, those athletes who run seasonally on hard or artificial playing surfaces as in soccer, football, field hockey, etc., would notice a need to spend more time maintaining inner thigh (adductor muscle) extensibility to avoid groin pulls… whereas the distance runner would recognize calves, hamstring muscles, and low back as areas requiring additional emphasis. This extra attention is applied during cooldown.

Gymnasts and dancers universally recognize the need to pursue flexibility full time. They constantly are flirting with injuries and will not risk, nor can they afford, the higher odds against them if they are not superbly flexible. Should it be any less so in other sports? You can not convince the authors that incomplete flexibility and less than full range of joint motion is in the best interest of the athlete or any individual.

Experienced athletes have learned their training programs through trial and error. This manual is intended to spare you some of the unnecessary suffering and disappointments these athletes have endured. By following the procedures as presented, you will find that the majority of injuries are avoidable and certainly should not be excused as accidental.

It must be understood that being superbly flexible is not the only goal. The athlete who is flexible but ignores the other components of physical fitness – **body structure, body composition, cardiorespiratory endurance, muscle power, muscle strength, muscle endurance** – will not enhance his or her performance. Therefore, accept **flexibility** as *one* important component in the prevention of athletic injuries through total fitness. The notable flexibility of gymnasts and dancers should not discourage you but should indicate in some cases the maximums which can be achieved. Each sport or work activity has its own peculiar characteristics and demands it places on the body. It should be remembered that the exercises, as presented, apply to your whole body, and your neuromuscu-

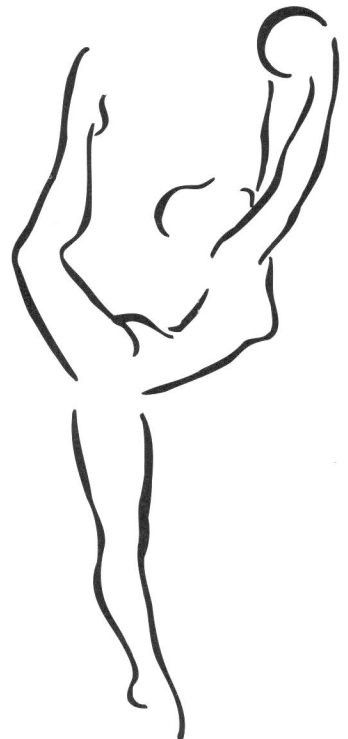

loskeletal responses to daily activity determine the body areas which should receive the most attention. Once you have achieved a high level of flexibility, it will be easier to maintain, and it will contribute greatly to make all forms of exercise beneficial, satisfying, and safe.

As you watch sports on TV, sometimes in slow motion replay, imagine the forces exerted by and on the moving structures of the body. Consider joint motions, muscle contractions, and– of equal importance – muscle relaxations (decelerations). Consider, also, the forces exerted on the body by the playing surface, other athletes, and implements of the game. Imagine the stresses and marvel at the human body's resilience.

You should learn as much about your body as possible – not abuse it unnecessarily, but take care of it. Your body will reward you for your efforts.

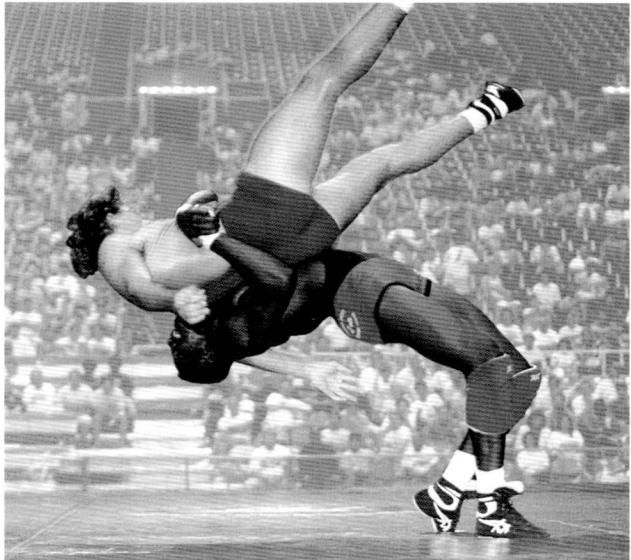

# CONCEPTS

We now present some simplified neuro-physiological concepts, their significance to flexibility, and their application to the methods which we have developed.

One readily can determine inflexibility to be the result of inactivity. In performing stretching techniques, care must be taken to prevent reactions which might result in soreness, followed by reluctance to use those body parts involved, and thence inactivity. Immobilization and reduced flexibility also will follow injuries to a greater or lesser degree. A more fit individual will recover more rapidly from injury, but it might be argued that the desire for fitness has led to those activities which have caused the injury in the first place. The pleasures of sports, or the level of fitness which provides satisfaction beyond just getting through the day, should dispel that argument and should encourage us to maintain ourselves better. Something has been lacking. Few who have been either active or inactive have been exposed to the benefits of a logical and well-constructed fitness program. It starts with mobility.

Stretching never has been fun and we do not dare to advance the notion that it is. The poor results achieved by methods using force have contributed to this. However, those who have used "active" stretching have been pleased with their success. It consumes little time and energy and requires no apparatus. Such a sensible do-it-yourself method will benefit you in sports and ordinary activities. Citing facts will inspire few to action, but it is necessary to present a few basic concepts which explain the reasoning behind our approach. Your success will be our satisfaction.

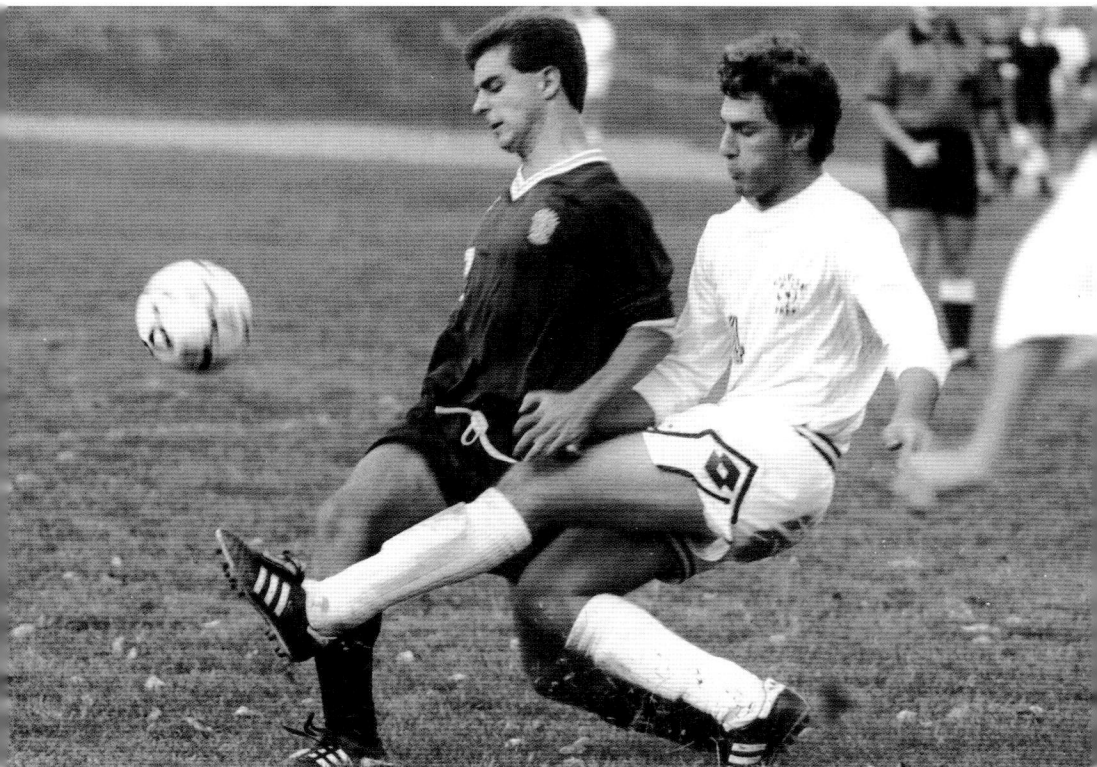

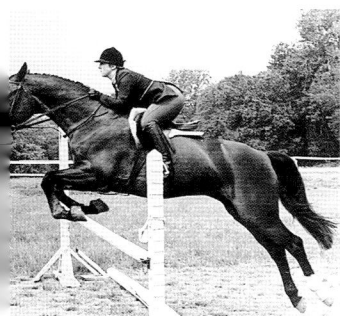

Because we break with traditional practices, it is permissible to say that our method is new. However, reciprocal innervation, from which we derive our method, is as ancient as motion itself. Applying this mechanism is a humbling experience because, like most things, it has been under our noses for so long. The scientific principles have been applied knowingly in some cases and unwittingly in others for a couple of generations. The principle of reciprocal innervation was described in Sir Charles Sherrington's work in 1904. It is simple but a marvel to contemplate in human or other animal neuromuscular function.

The natural reciprocal process of your nervous system used in "active" stretching allows several things to make it a safe and effective method. "Active" stretching eliminates all of the problems caused by passive, forced stretching. Once the principle is appreciated, anyone can reason out "active" applications with confidence.

If you never have applied "active" stretching in our total approach method, our following statement might annoy you: No individual should be stretched passively, i.e., forcefully, except by an athletic trainer or physical therapist for therapeutic purposes.

Utilizing reciprocal innervation in flexibility training permits and demands a whole new way of thinking. Most of the ill-founded principles and limitations of passive (static) stretching can and must be ignored in order to derive the benefits of this "new" method. You soon will wonder why traditional stretching, with its drawbacks, has persisted for so long.

It is the common assumption that all stretching is the same, but as one by one, traditional bouncing, static and forced stretching, dangerous body positions, etc. are debunked, you will find pre-warmup "active" stretching to be most effective and safe. "Active" stretching in our

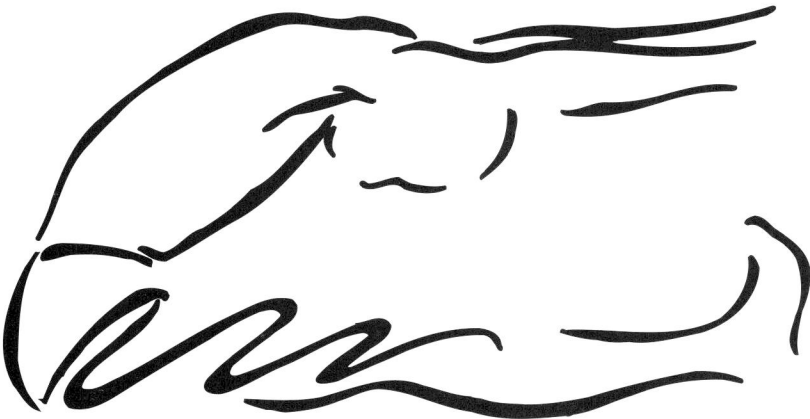

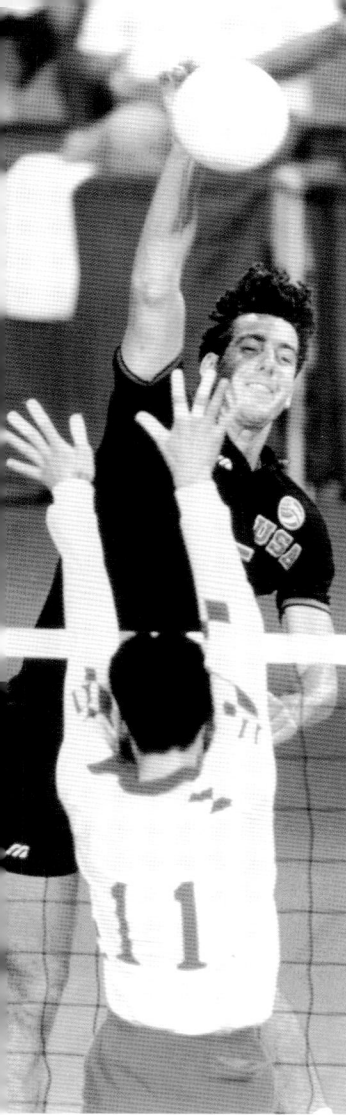

terms relies upon the interaction of *agonist* and *antagonist* muscles. This is to say: When one muscle or group of muscles (agonist) contracts, the opposing one (antagonist) relaxes under neurological control. Under normal conditions we are not aware of this neurological function, but we can imagine how stiff, or motionless, we would be without it. The reciprocally innervated neuromuscular system is in place and performing its function. *Utilize it*. As you develop your body awareness, you will sense the "active" components in every stretching technique employed.

Some muscle activities in work or play are prolonged and/or performed with so much force that normally balanced interaction among muscles, their condition, and tone can be upset. This results in muscle shortening without full relaxation when the activity is terminated. No doubt we all have experienced the good feeling of muscle tiredness. We also know the pain and spasm associated with injury from (1) the loss of coordination from fatigue or (2) overextensibility of muscles and tendons – the two causes of muscle strain. This type of soft tissue injury can be prolonged and disabling if not cared for immediately and properly. Prevention is preferred. A total method, under the control of the individual and no one else, is most sensible. Where but on the playing or practice field should we expect someone else to exert undue forces upon our bodies?

The matter of pain (not of disease origin) must be considered. Pain is a warning to be heeded for safety. If there is muscular pain as the result of injury, you must combine your judgment with that of a physical therapist or athletic trainer for therapeutic application of stretching – sometimes of a quite different form. Such circumstances support our proposal that "active" stretching be performed every day for prevention – avoiding need for therapeutic measures.

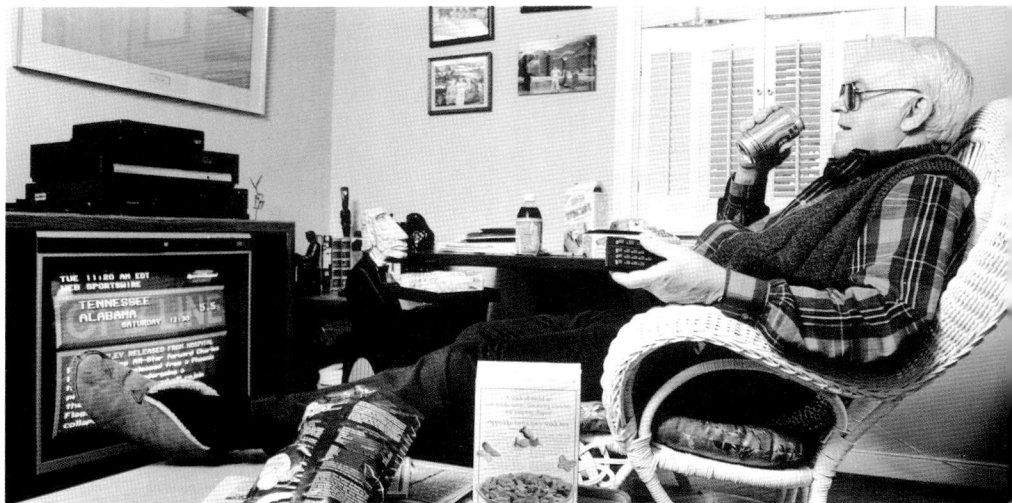

The relative inactivity of the sedentary or improperly exercised individual results in subtle shortening of the more powerful muscles followed by an insidious reduction in the range of motion of the joints upon which the muscles act. An individual who is in this state, and who performs a sudden movement, surely is subjecting himself or herself to increased chances of injury.

Following your "active" stretching, it is important to warm up thoroughly. Warmup is the gradual increase in mobility of body parts, joints, and muscles through careful repetitive motions. When there are delays between athletic events, it is wise to retain the body heat which your muscles have generated by using proper clothing. Provided you have gone through a balanced warmup with emphasis upon specific muscles required by your sport, your warmup is adequate when there is the appearance of perspiration upon your brow. This indicates, generally, a rise in core (rectal) temperature of 2 to 3 degrees F which can last 45 minutes or longer.

To digress a bit further into the important area of warmups, they also have been considered passive or active. Some athletes have experimented with passive heating for their warmup preceding sports participation. This has ranged from localized heating with a hot pack to generalized heating in a sauna bath. It has been borne out that the body's physiological responses to the stress of outside heating are not genuine or as efficient as the internal heating which is the body's active byproduct of work metabolism. It seems logical that the sweat on your brow, indicating a proper warmup, should be achieved legitimately through body movements common to the impending athletic performance.

It is equally important to perform the reverse process and cool down after activities. This is a good time to stretch again those areas which you have found to pose the greatest tendency toward tightness. Your body already has been warmed up thoroughly, and your blood has been directed to the active muscles to meet their demand. A sudden cessation of activity leaves the blood stranded or pooled in these areas. Cooling down facilitates the return of blood to the brain, to the intestinal tract, and to the heart.

Traditional methods support a physioogical view that some body warmth derived from gentle motion beforehand enhances static stretching. This seems to be true. However, we don't promote static stretching because it is neurophysiologically wrong. High numbers of injuries, occurring during warmups and practice sessions, persist. We question such methods which are supposed to prevent injuries and improve performance but don't. In actual practice we find that few athletes initiate their warmup and then interrupt it to perform adequate static stretching. They tend to continue the warmup and neglect the stretching entirely, or they perform the stretching hurriedly (perhaps ballistically) and incompletely. Also, should the athletes partially warm up and then stretch thoroughly (up to 30 minutes), they will find themselves cooling down. Then they will have to warm up again – perhaps inadequately. The warmup is too important to be treated in this manner. Contrary to their intuitions, their stretching exercises have become lost in their warmup, increasing rather than decreasing their risk of injury. We believe that our "active" method, which is physiologically normal, provides a slight warming effect to muscles. We could not detect any increase in core temperature, however, supporting our contention that it be utilized as pre-warmup followed by warmup.

The most successful example of stretching before warmup is the gymnast who will do nothing until he or she has stretched – slowly and methodically. Then he or she does basic warmup passes or moves on the apparatus. Because there is considerable cooling down between events and individual performances, there are warmup periods on each piece of apparatus between events. You will see the gymnast stretching preceding these warmups and again immediately before his or her individual performance. These are unusual circumstances, but we feel that no athlete should be less dedicated to his or her body's needs when performance and safety are the desired end. The gymnast who uses "active" stretching between events will shorten the time to maintain or regain flexibility lost during these unavoidable periods of cooling.

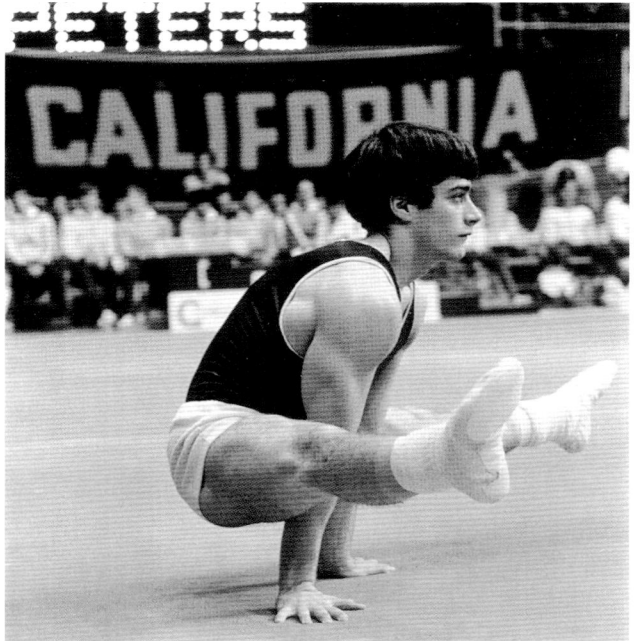

With adequate explanation, individuals are also motivated to apply this performance discipline in a team situation. Players of a local high school soccer coach (utilizing our program since 1978) have not missed a single practice or game as a result of a non-contact muscle injury. We have been working closely with an increasing number of high school and college soccer teams whose every practice and game is preceded by a 20 plus-minute "active" stretching program. The only injuries have been those related to trauma or direct contact.

We are heartened by the broad applicability of this method, and know that any dedicated individual can benefit. Although we appear to address ourselves to the needs of the athlete, be assured that we equally recognize the needs of the nonathlete who stretches solely for mobility. Only the goal, not the level of importance, differs. As a nonathlete or athlete, you are stretching to meet the rigors of a day's work or sporting event. Motion enhances circulation and most of our body heat comes from muscle contraction. Therefore, it is understandable that body temperature is lower in the morning. Whether you stretch early or at different times of the day, equal precautions prevail in performing the exercises.

Another note of interest is that individuals in our Sports Kinetics programs are not handed a sheet of instructions but are led personally through all of the flexibility procedures until they understand each one and its purpose. This is one reason we have produced the video "FLEXIBILITY SETS YOU FREE!" and have taken so much care with the instructions and their accompanying photographs in THE FLEXIBILITY MANUAL. We sincerely want everyone to know the what, how, when, and why of maintaining flexibility and its importance.

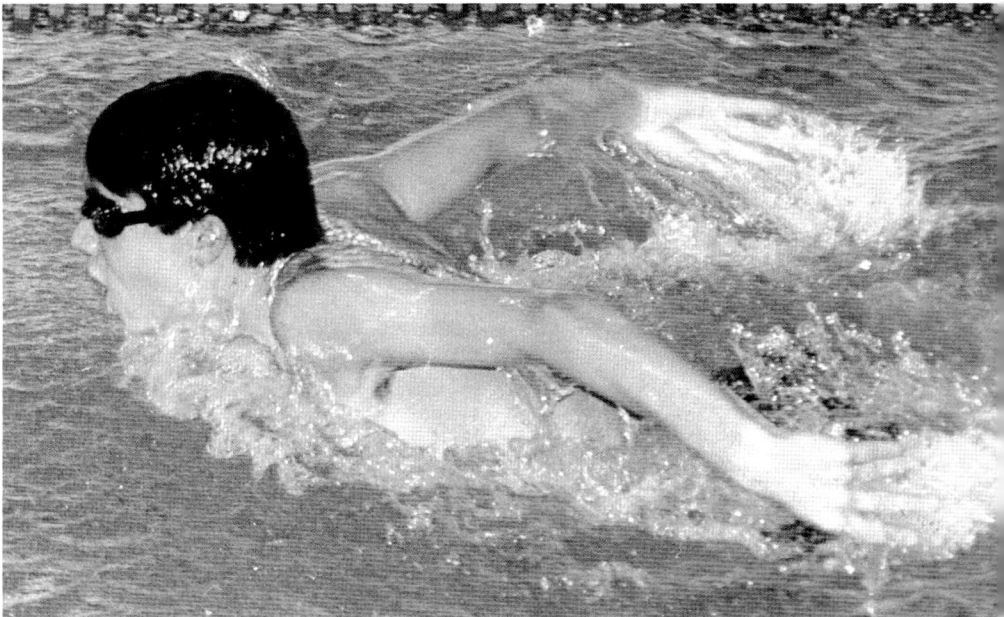

# STRETCH REFLEXES

Stretch reflexes are the contractile responses of muscles which are stretched. As normal functions, they act as protective responses to sudden demands placed upon muscles.

If one had to rely solely on visual assessment of the effect of a weight being placed in one's hand, conscious awareness by the brain most likely would take too long to contract the muscles needed to hold the weight steady. The weight would drop with a force that could tear restricting muscle and perhaps even joint structures. Suppose you close your eyes to eliminate anticipation. The unconscious, normal reflex action to the same sudden stretch results in a muscular contraction quick enough to prevent full descent of the weight. The reflex has prevented injury. In sports or work activity, if the force is so great that it exceeds the muscle's ability to decelerate motion successfully, the muscle will be torn and possibly the joint structure will be injured also.

In stretching you want to discourage stimulation of the stretch reflex. You must enter each position slowly and stretch very slowly in order to minimize the frequency of impulses from the muscle which cause a neuromuscular response. Although discharges continue as long as the muscle is stretched, a slow and steady tension will permit greater adaptation with less undesirable (for your purpose) muscle shortening, and lengthening of the muscles can be achieved more easily. Bouncing while stretching can be self-defeating because it stimulates stretch reflexes. Our observations have indicated that the lengthening of muscle in a ballistic manner is not as enduring as when performed with a slow stretch— preferably "active."

Static stretching also causes an increase in unwanted neuromuscular response, although more subtly. The muscle, sensing potential injury, tends to contract and takes a prolonged period of time to relax. Whereas, with "active" methods, which utilize the neuromechanism of reciprocal innervation, resultant inhibition is instantaneous.

With "active" stretching, you reach to take up the slack, hold the contraction, but ease up enough to avoid pain. After allowing 10 to 15 seconds of adaptation, you should be able to reach a bit farther the next time. The reason to avoid pain is self-evident. Pain tells you to stop. If not, motion will be terminated in a more drastic manner by injury or muscle spasm, either one interfering with your intended goal of increasing your flexibility.

# IMMOBILIZATION AND INACTIVITY

We know the ravages of loss of function following severe trauma to the body. Pain and swelling are a defensive and protective consequence of accidental or surgical insult. Extent of tissue injury and degree of tissue repair affect function to varying degrees. The DeMarlais Tables[1] serve to indicate the negative effects of immobilization – especially on the joints:

It takes three days for recovery for each day the knee is immobilized. The shoulder, if it is not immobilized after injury, will regain full range of motion in 18 days. If it is immobilized for one week, it will take 52 days; two weeks will take 121 days; three weeks will take 300 days. These effects are disastrous.

1. Origin of the De Marlais Tables eludes us. Any information would be appreciated.

Immobilization jeopardizes the balance of fluid and collagen fibers, which are a major part of the structural network of connective tissues. In the photographs, the dark-stained collagen fibers appear among the lighter fat and noncollagenous connective tissues. They present varying degrees of apparent disorganization in different areas of the body. Notice their density and alignment, aquired through function, reflecting the toughness of the Achilles tendon (heel cord) in specimen #1. Compare this with their random appearance in less dense subcutaneous tissue, specimen #2.

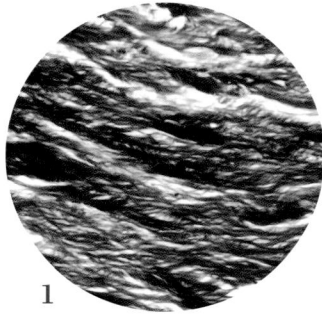

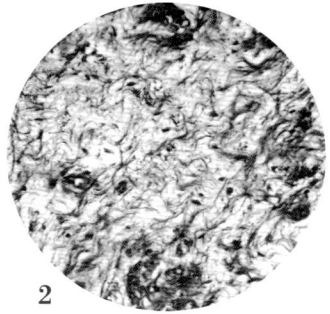

Connective tissue is undergoing continuous replacement 24 hours a day. If it is not stretched, the collagen meshwork within it is reorganized into a shortened state, and loss of motion results.

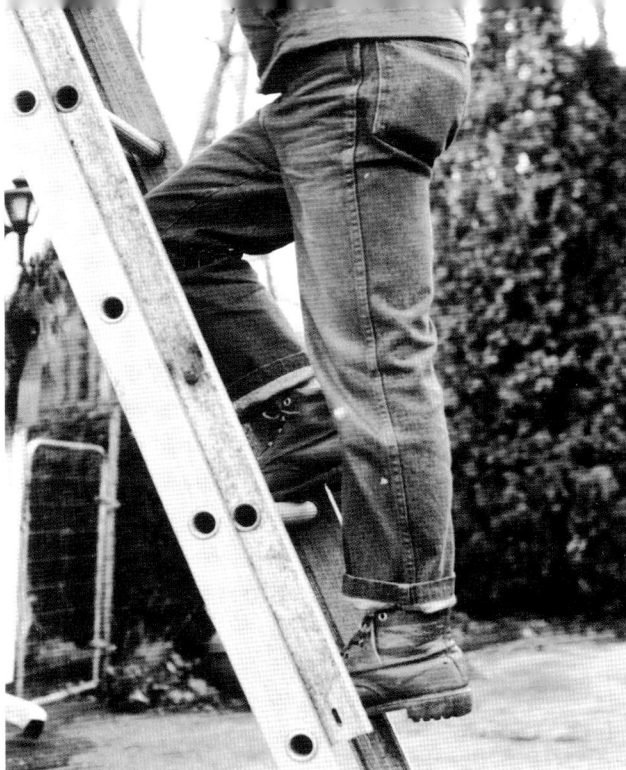

# MOTION

Muscles serve not only to activate motion (agonists) but opposing (antagonist) groups also serve to restrain motion. In flexion, not only must flexors contract but the extensors must relax proportionally. In extension, the extensors contract, and the flexors must relax (reciprocal innervation). Thus, motion is dependent upon several factors:

1. The contraction of the agonists
2. The graded relaxation of the antagonists
3. The normal tonicity of the ligamentous structures
4. The normal joint structures
5. The lubrication by synovial fluid within the joint capsule.

Muscles also serve an additional function in support. Although standing is thought to be motionless, there is an almost imperceptible interplay of agonist and antagonist muscles which balance the whole body. During sports or other activities, this reciprocal innervation process prevents overaction of muscle groups and permits fineness or skill with which a movement can be executed (coordination).

We now consider a theory of the elastic behavior of muscle in storing spring-like tension. The length of a muscle at the time it is called on to contract influences the magnitude of its contraction. That is, within physiological limits, a stretched muscle contracts more forcefully than when it is unstretched at the time of its activation. Liken the pre-jump position of a human to the preliminary crouch of an animal of prey. There is a decided dynamic "wind-up" or pre-tension placed on the muscles which will impart additional and more effective energy release. If this optimum position or "set" cannot be assumed, owing to the effects of inflexibility or for some other limiting reason, performance suffers. Therefore, we would like to have available the maximum "wind-up" provided by complete flexibility. Of course, we also would like to have a "follow-through", unrestricted by muscle tightness and/or limited joint range of motion, to prevent injury.

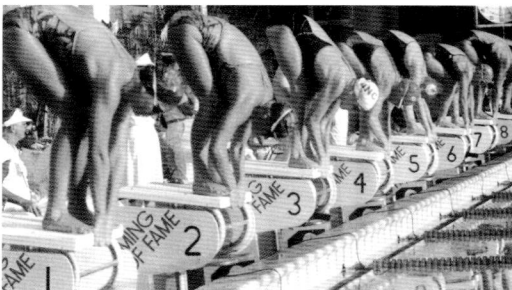
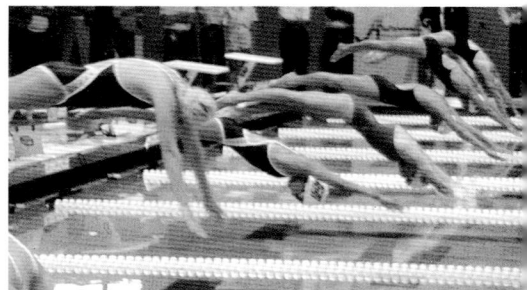

# FLEXIBILITY PROGRAM

## BEFORE YOU BEGIN

Generally, it is accepted that approximately 80% of all back pain cases are related to underexercise. More medical observers agree that inactivity (hypokinesis) results in muscular imbalance, structural change, and pain. Exercise should be selective and not a quick assumption or resumption of physical activity following inactive periods. Exercise in itself is not the cure-all for back pain or any other musculoskeletal disability. You must gain the optimum flexibility, warm up, exercise in the proper manner and intensity, and follow your activity with cooling down.

Everyone probably has muscle strength and functional imbalances derived from athletic, occupational, or sedentary activities and inactivities. Previous injuries, also, can result in uncorrected limitations of joint ranges of motion. What is normal? How flexible should a normal joint be? We know what is desirable, and we have standardized orthopedic measurements, but allowances have to be made for the "double-jointed," certain sports requirements, and previously injured body structures. Some circles express concern regarding overstretching which could result in hypermobility and instability of the joints, contributing to injury. We see this in the dance/ballet community. "Active" stretching, however, is *self-limiting*. It utilizes only self-administered, controlled, agonist muscle contractions which cannot overstretch the antagonist muscle or other healthy joint structures.

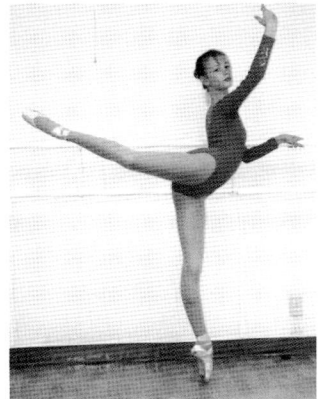

In some flexibility positions, you will be stretching more than one area effectively. However, most positions depicted are isolated in order to provide protection through awareness and control of the muscles being stretched. Functionally, few body structures move without being in concert with others, and a combined motion might have a defective component which could be the unsuspected cause of an injury. By isolating the muscles you can detect potential problems better. The slowness and non-ballistic nature of "active" stretching aids in this also.

# SOME IMPORTANT DO'S AND DON'TS

Don't just open THE FLEXIBILITY MANUAL and start. Look at the pictures in sequence and the areas being stretched. Read the accompanying instructions beforehand, and analyze each picture for body alignment and position of feet and hands. Try to visualize in advance how you will position yourself in the same manner as the photographed subject. You will learn more quickly. Carefully read Considerations (p. 73). If you don't prevent mistakes at the start, you may never recognize them later.

As you follow the sequence of photographs, you occasionally will notice an optional position photograph. Such exercises are progressive. When you are satisfied that you are performing the first exercise with ease, try the next position. Then, this will be your new sequence. If it doesn't feel right, don't hesitate to return to the previous one. Try again at a future time. You won't benefit at all by rushing the procedure. It's how you do the exercises that will produce results, not just doing them. We have presented a number of reasons for maintaining the integrity of your muscles and the joint structures about which they function. We feel strongly that the success you achieve will depend on regularity of application. Set aside a few minutes each day learning and performing the method in its presented sequence.

Depending on your general condition and activities you pursue, some exercise positions may present little or no challenge. Others may seem impossible and discouraging. If so, return to the explanations of our concepts, weigh the benefits, and resume with calculated determination. If you experience any sensation other than that of ordinary muscle stretch, don't persist. Also, some individuals may have pre-existing conditions which should not be aggravated. "Listen" to your body. Skip those exercise positions until they can benefit you.

Your having obtained THE FLEXIBILITY MANUAL indicates your interest level is high and that you recognize the need for flexibility. So that you are not testing your human weaknesses everyday, it is wise to plan a firm time of day, each day, that you are going to do your flexibility program (perhaps while you are watching television). This will eliminate a daily battle with your conscience, and you will be well on your productive way. Success, a good motivator, is not imme-

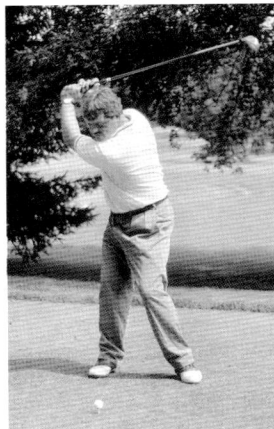

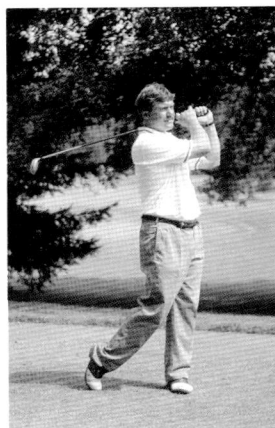

diate, nor does motivation come easily for many of us. A change in mind set may take ten minutes before you become engrossed in a new activity. Allowing for this should help you to combat procrastination.

Although we are able to guide a beginner through the entire flexibility program in about 30 minutes, it will take you longer to read the instructions, analyze the pictures, and apply the exercises. To make the learning process more manageable, first obtain a general idea of the program by relating all of the instructions to all of the pictures. Perform only a few exercises for a couple of days. Then proceed to a few more exercises after repeating the previous ones, and so on. By starting at the beginning each day, you will reinforce the previous material as you are learning the next. Within a couple of weeks you will know the whole program thoroughly and in proper sequence. As your flexibility improves and is maintained, the time required will decrease accordingly. Then it may take you only about 20 minutes.

Do every exercise which doesn't hurt or otherwise present risk. This is your daily "systems check" of your whole body. It is your time to detect any adverse changes and to deal with them immediately. If you are satisfied with your flexibility in a particular position, you may skip that one. Now to work! Remove jewelry, chewing gum, etc. (as you should for all sports). Wear loose clothing, especially about the neck and waist. Shoes are not necessary until you stretch your heel cords in the standing position. Then your arches should have the benefit of their support as well as any orthotic inserts which you normally use.

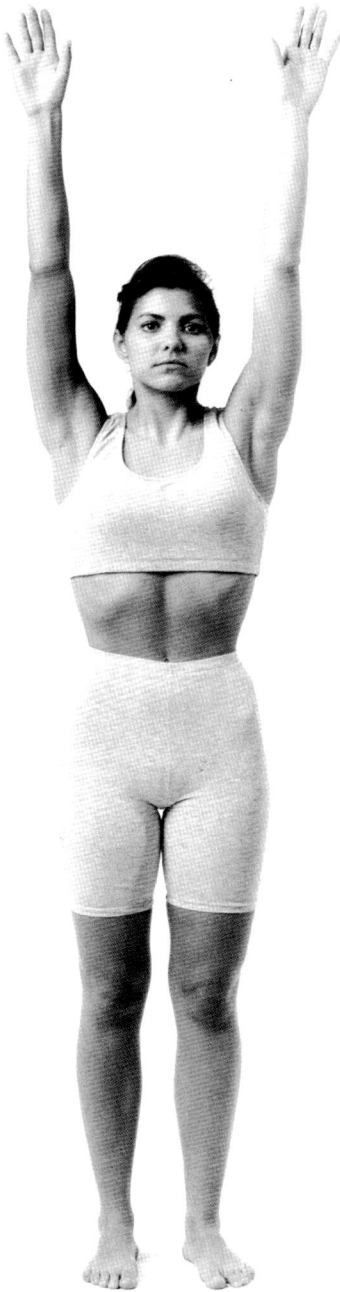

Reach arms over head, elevating your shoulders at the same time.

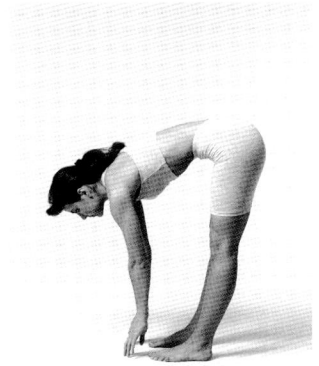

While maintaining this stretch, reach toward the floor, contracting your abdominal and hip flexor muscles. Keep your knees straight. Don't bounce to get there.

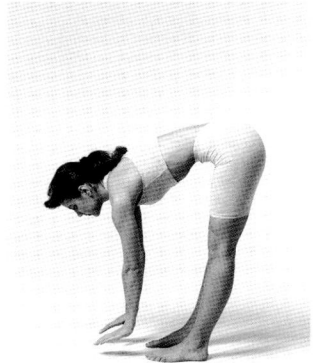

# 1 REACHING - Ceiling to floor

To Determine Your Initial Mobility

3 REPETITIONS

NOTE: If successful in touching the floor (an accepted average), extend your wrists to stretch your forearm flexors.

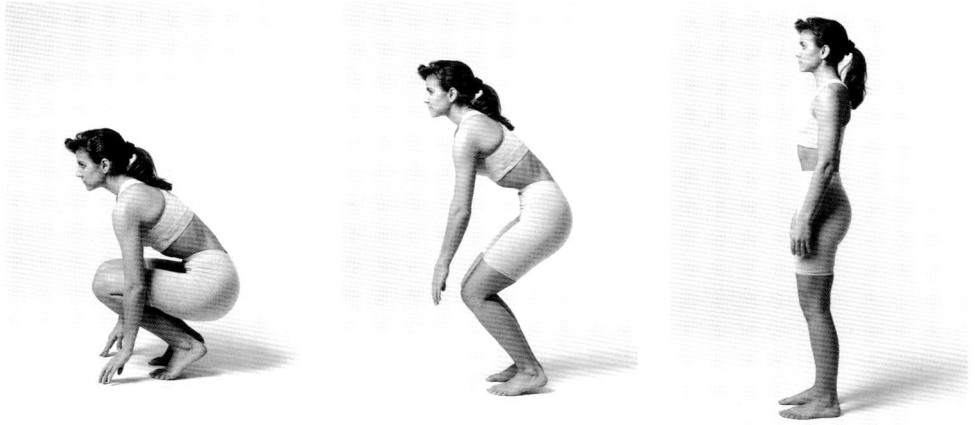

Bend your knees, using your legs to rise, in order to protect your back.

NOTE: Consider this protective measure during your daily work activities.

# 2 REACHING - Supine

To Align the Spine

## 1 REPETITION  Hold 10 seconds.

Stretch arms overhead. Align spine by "walking" heels away from fingertips. This is quite relaxing, and you might find yourself yawning, which is an active stretch of the jaw and other muscles.

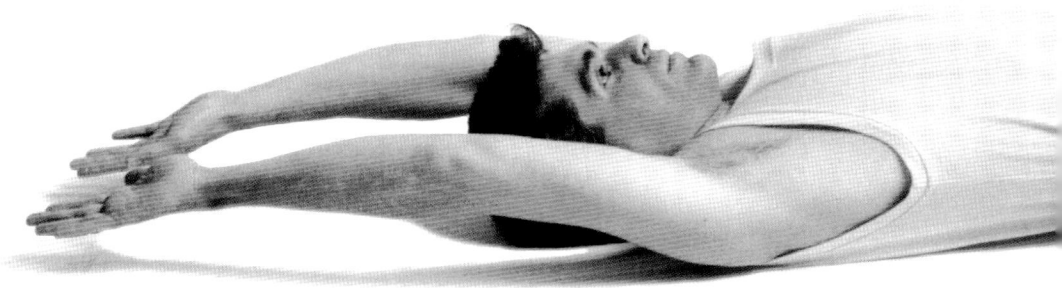

# 3 BREATHING - Abdominal

For relaxation

## 3 REPETITIONS

Knees bent, arms at sides, and hands half on abdomen and half on rib cage.

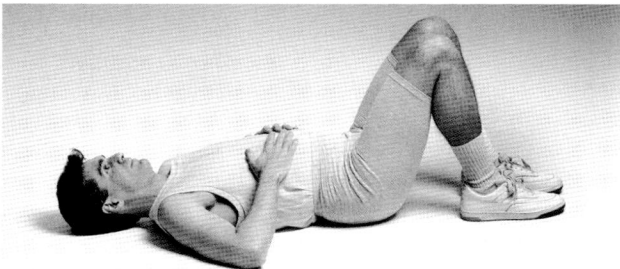

Inhale abdominally, activating your diaphragm, in a relaxed manner. There should be no motion of the rib cage.

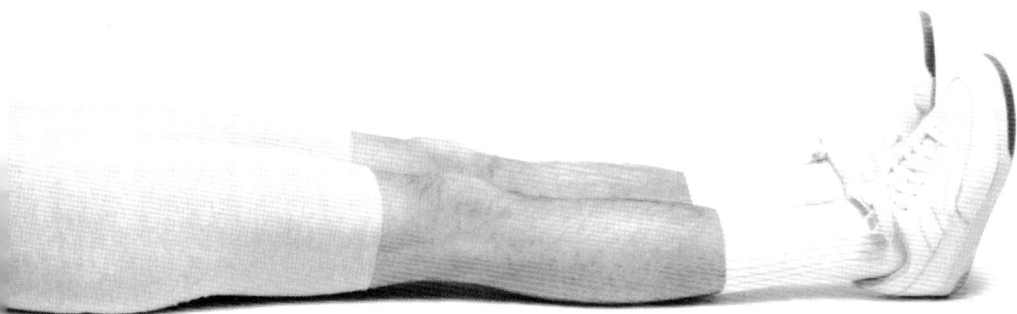

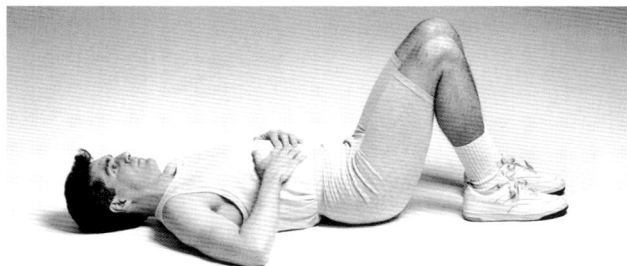

You should feel your abdomen rise on inhalation and fall on exhalation with no motion of the rib cage. You will be aware of air entering and leaving your nasal passages as you breathe.

# 4 BREATHING - Abdomen to Chest

To Mobilize the Rib Cage

## 3 REPETITIONS

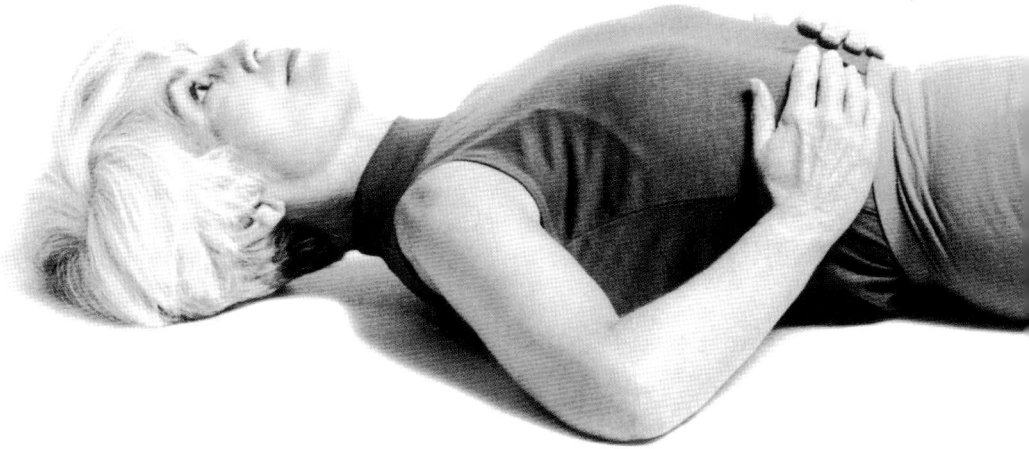

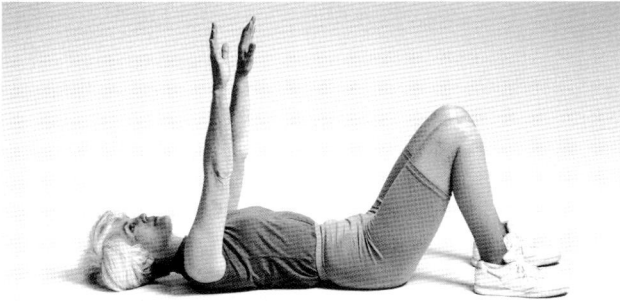

Start with abdominal breathing. Then raise arms overhead and continue to pull air up into chest. You will be aware of a greater volume of air passing through your throat (pharynx).

NOTE: The abdominal (diaphragmatic) breathing, followed by chest excursion, enhances lung expansion by enlarging both the abdominal and chest cavities.

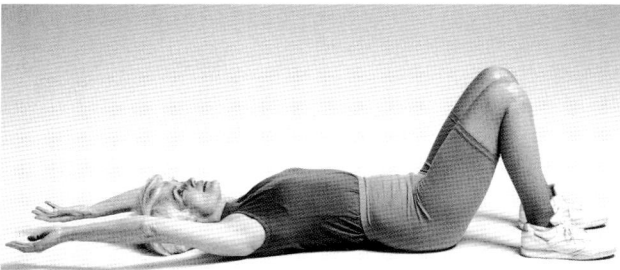

Arc arms down to sides as you...

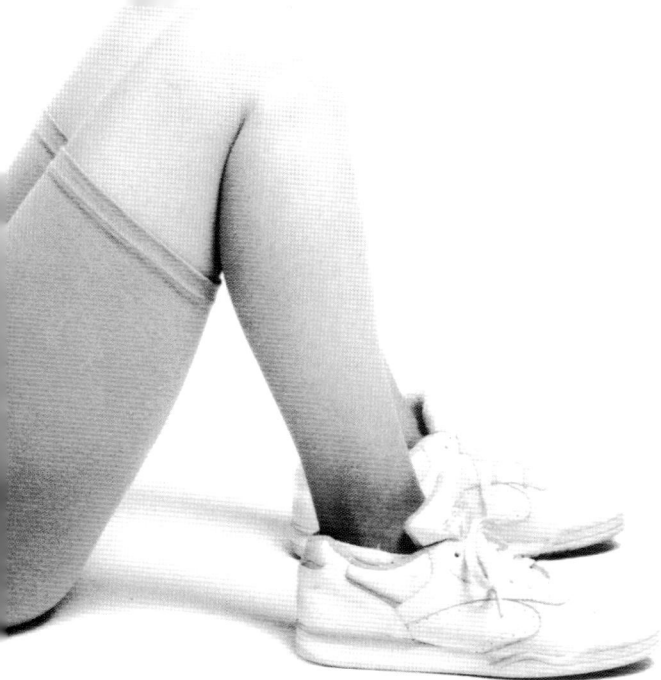

Exhale through your mouth with final forced exhalation to expel as much residual air as possible.

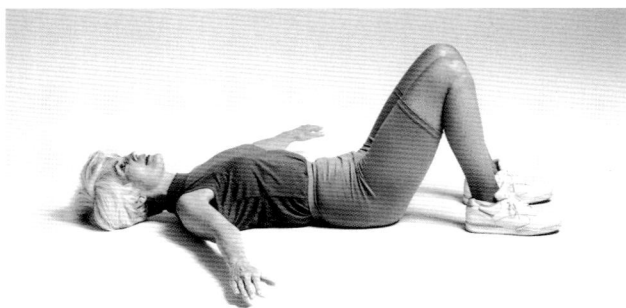

Repeat three times with restful breathing in between to prevent hyperventilation.

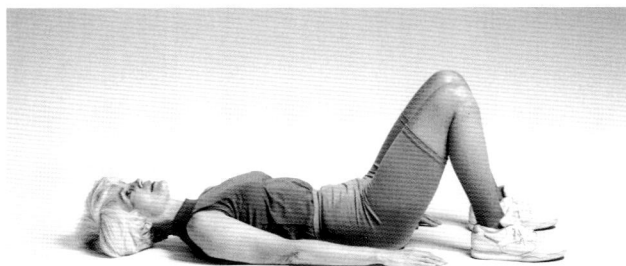

# 5 PELVIC TILT

**Low Back**

**3 REPETITIONS**

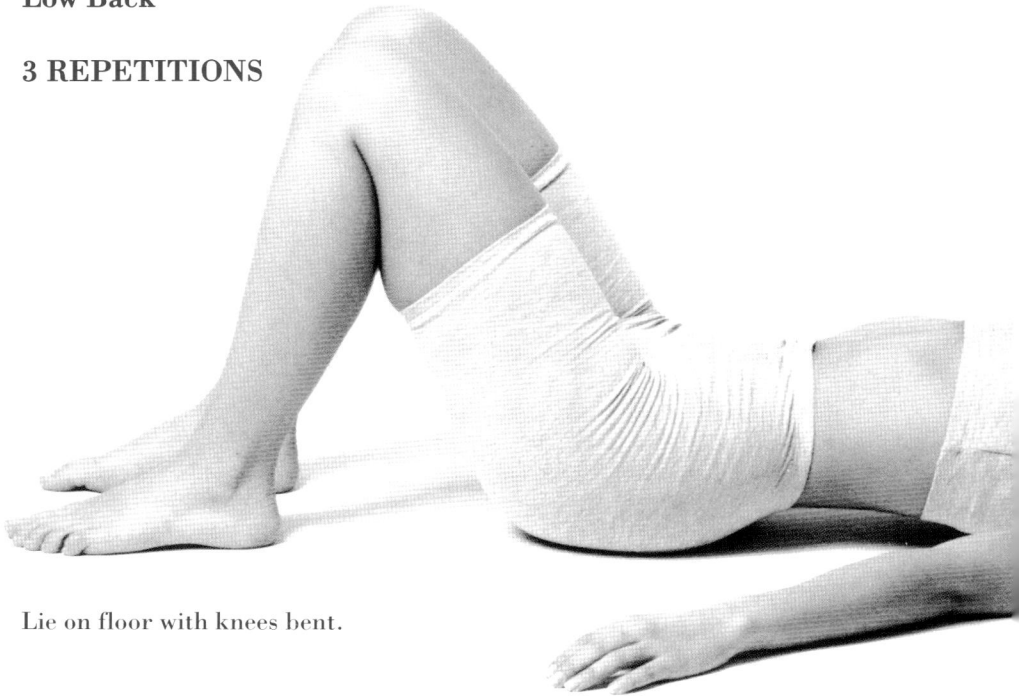

Lie on floor with knees bent.

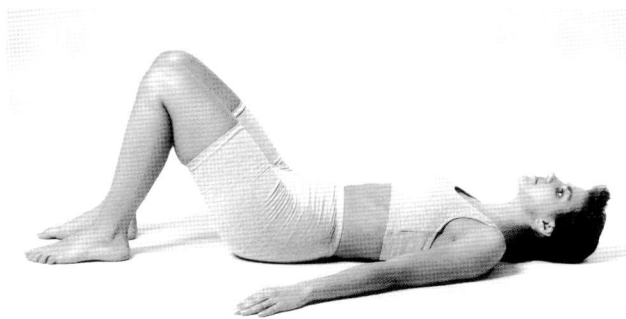

To flatten low back to floor, tilt pelvis upward by
contracting your abdominal muscles only. Do not
push down with feet. Do not hold your breath.
Hold 10 seconds.

# 6 PARTIAL SITUP

Back

## 3 REPETITIONS

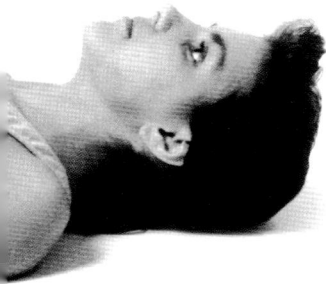

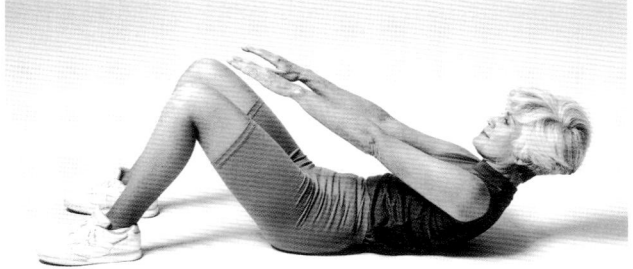

Knees bent, tilt your pelvis as in the previous exercise. Reach fingers to or beyond knees without touching them. Rise slowly.

Don't try to sit up all the way. Just maintain tension in your abdominal muscles for a count of 10 seconds. Do not hold your breath. Descend slowly.

NOTE: This is an excellent example of reciprocal innervation. While your abdominals are contracting, your opposing back muscles are relaxing.

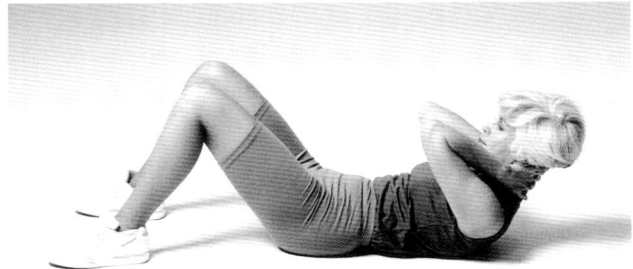

If you have a problem with your neck, clasp your hands behind your neck for support. If this does not help, postpone or skip this exercise.

# 7 ANKLE/CALF STRETCH

## 3 REPETITIONS each leg

Starting position: contract
front thigh muscles firmly to
keep knee straight.

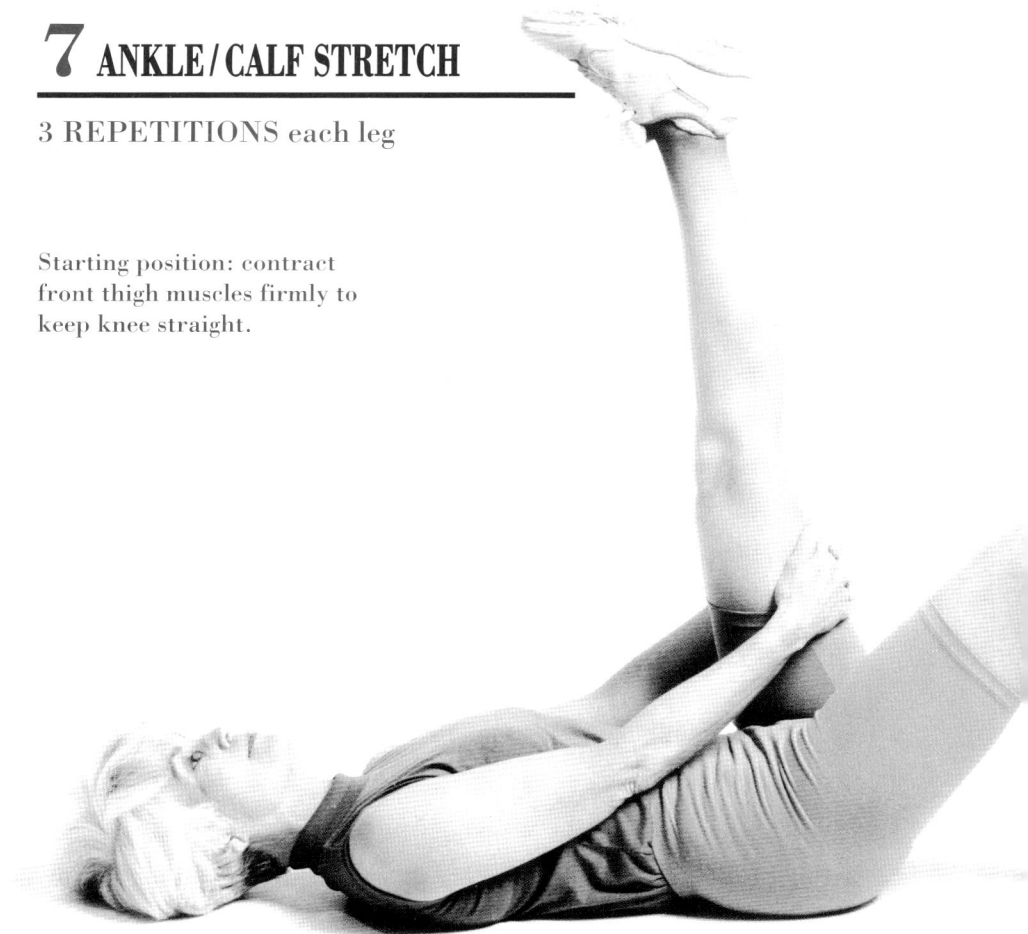

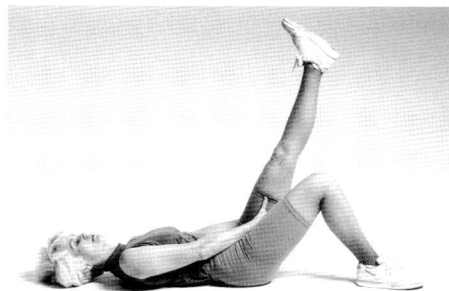

Optional position:
In order to keep your knee perfectly
straight, leg may be held at a lower
angle in the beginning. This is necessary to get proper stretch of the calf
muscles.

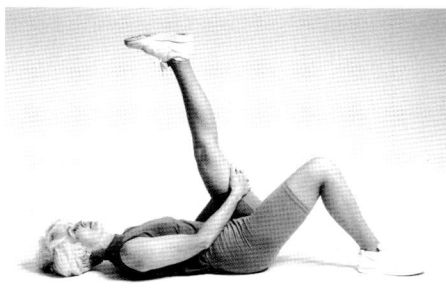

Optional position:
A more acute hip angle is desirable,
provided the knee of the supported
leg can be held straight to get proper
stretch of the calf muscles.

NOTE: Move slowly through these positions without
holding for the usual 10 seconds.

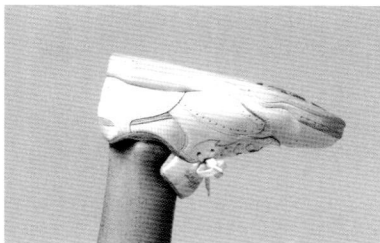

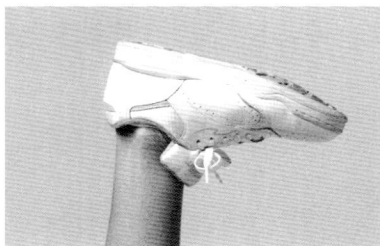

Pull toes
down toward
you.

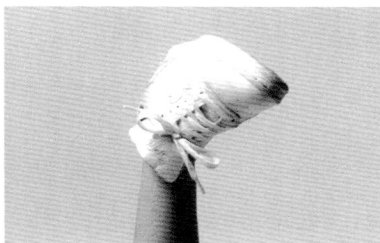

Turn
ankle in.

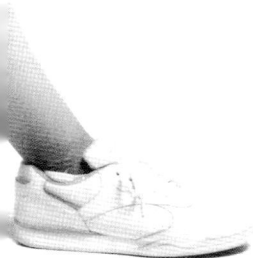

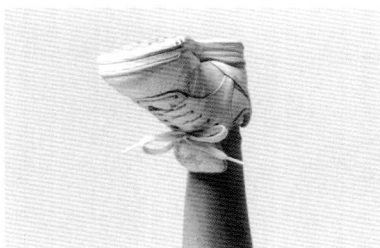

Turn ankle
out.

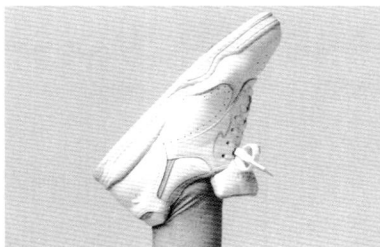

Point toes up.

Pull toes
down.

# 8 PLOUGH

Back and Hamstrings

3 REPETITIONS each leg

NOTE: This exercise is too strenuous for some individuals. It should not be incorporated if there is a back or neck problem.

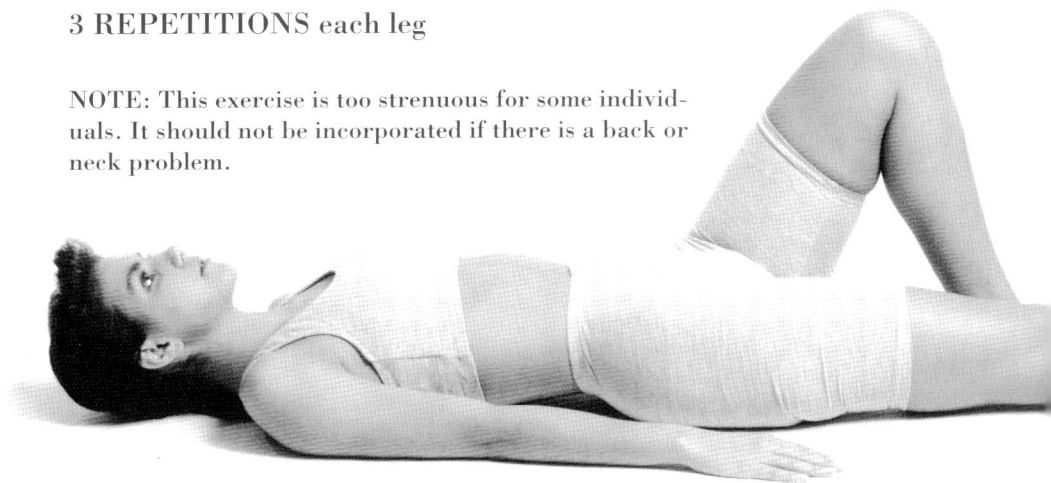

One leg bent with other on floor.

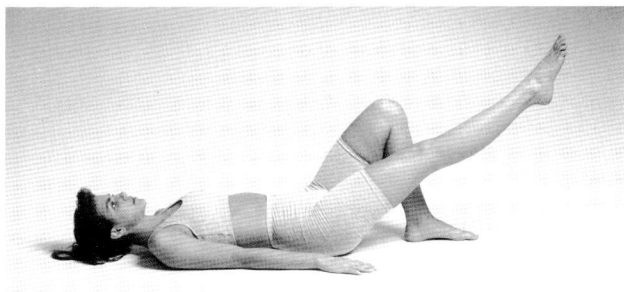

Slowly raise the straight leg to a 30° angle...

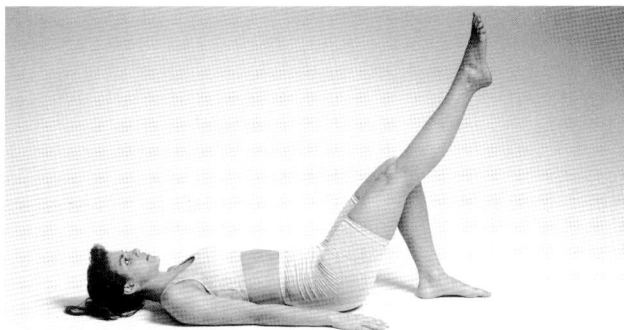

Then to a 60° angle...

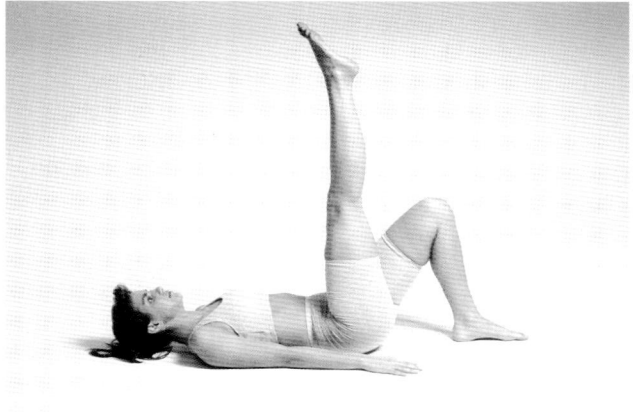

Finally to a 90° angle.

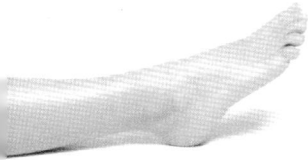

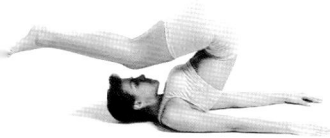

Optional position:
If back and legs are too
tight, allow knees to bend.

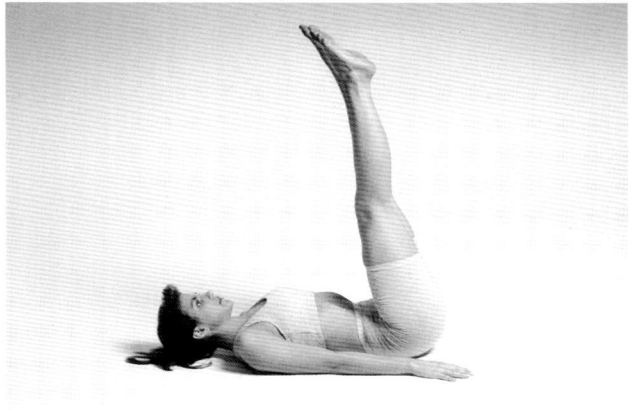

Raise the bent leg to 90 °.

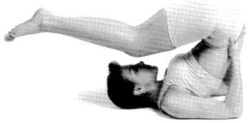

Optional position:
If you have difficulty, support hips with hands.

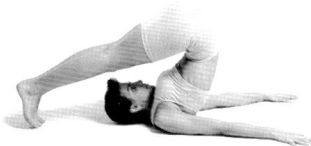

Optional position: If toes
touch floor readily with
knees straight, attempt to
pull toes toward your head
for increased calf muscle
stretch.

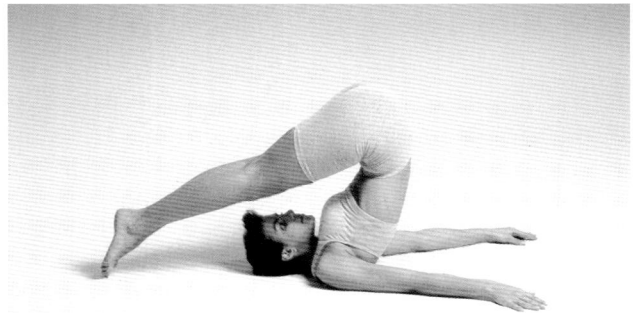

Slowly roll legs and hips overhead attempting to touch
floor with toes, preferably with both knees straight.
Hold for 10 seconds.

CONTINUED

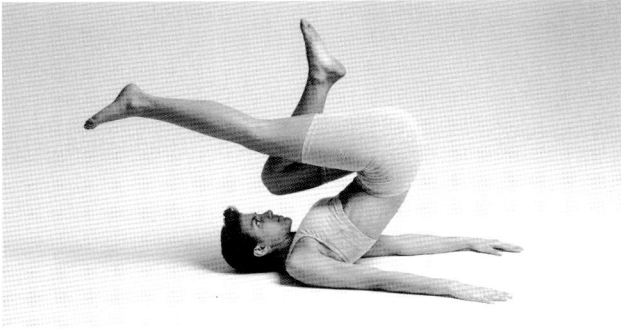

After bending the same leg, descend slowly.

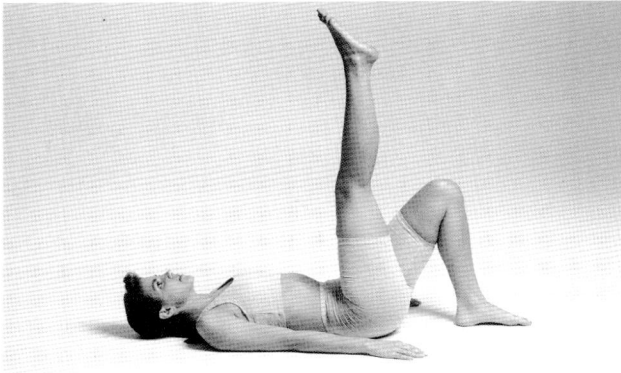

The bent leg should touch the floor before lowering the straight leg.

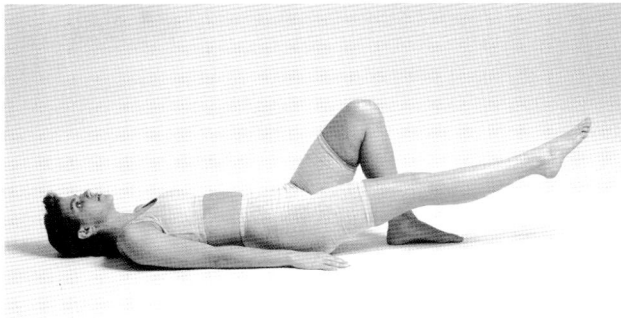

Lower the straight leg.
Repeat with other side.

# 9 BUTTERFLY

Adductors, Groin

## 3 REPETITIONS

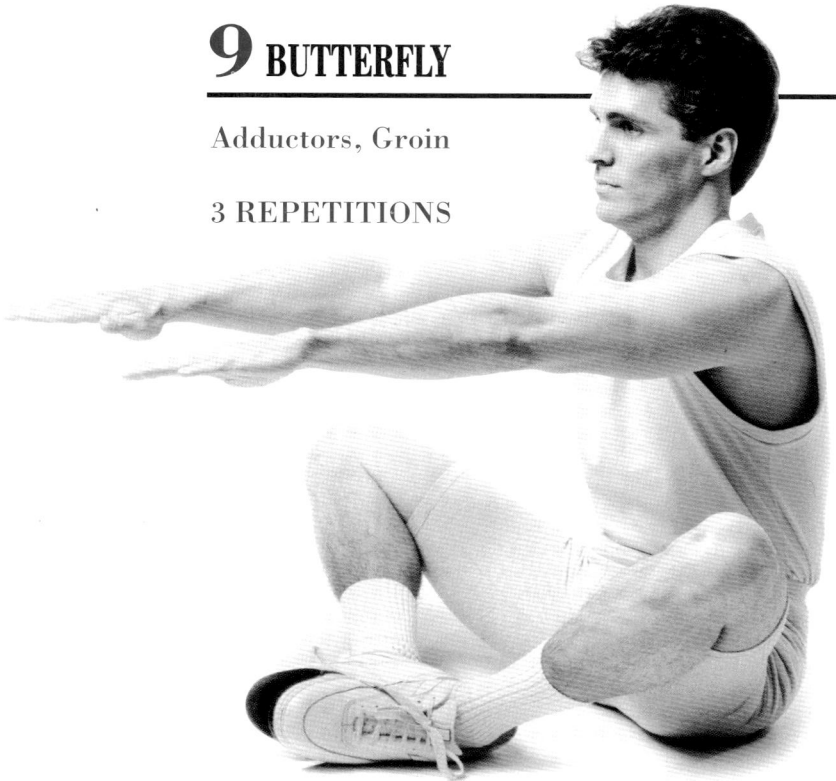

Soles of feet together, reach over toes with both hands. Reach short of discomfort, backing off a little if necessary, and hold for 10 seconds. Do not touch floor.

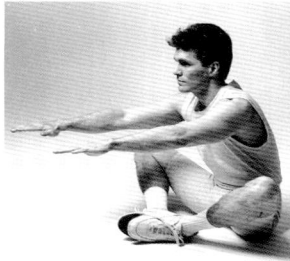

Try to reach your chest forward rather than your head which should be erect.

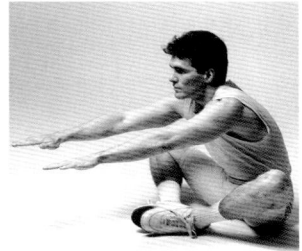

When fully forward, advance arms for additional stretch between your shoulder blades.

NOTE: Actively flare knees down toward floor for increased groin stretch.

45

# 10 STRADDLE

Adductors

## 3 REPETITIONS

Legs well apart with knees straight, reach straight forward short of discomfort, and hold for 10 seconds.
Do not touch floor.
Note: The stretch will be felt farther down the inside surfaces of both legs.

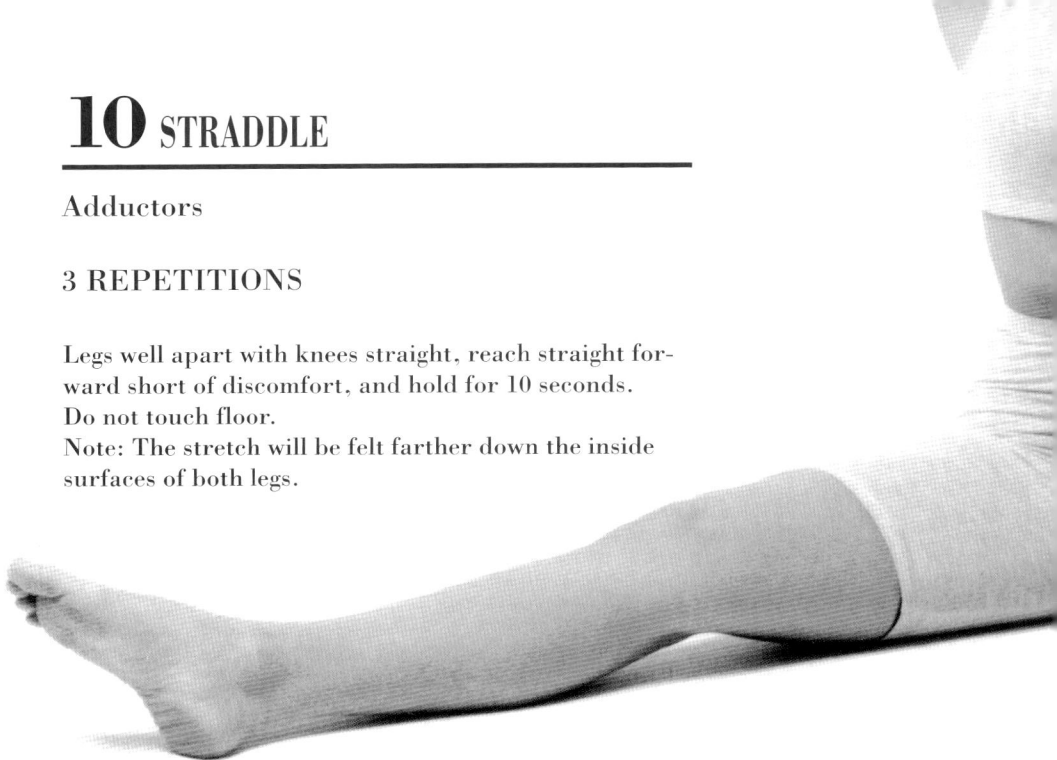

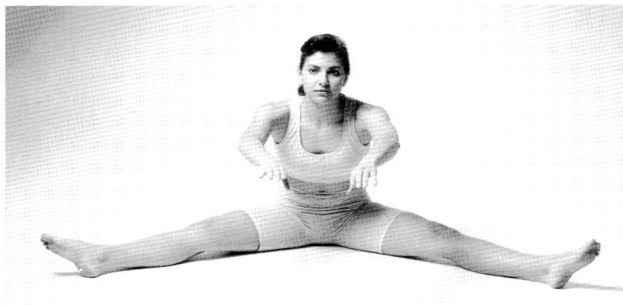

Keep head up, back straight without slouching.

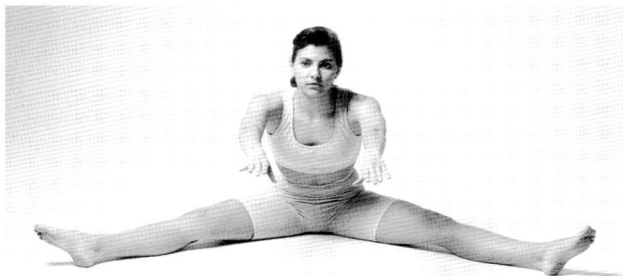

Advance your arms for additional stretch between your shoulder blades.

# 11 ONE HAND REACH ACROSS

Back, Hamstrings, Shoulders

3 REPETITIONS  each side

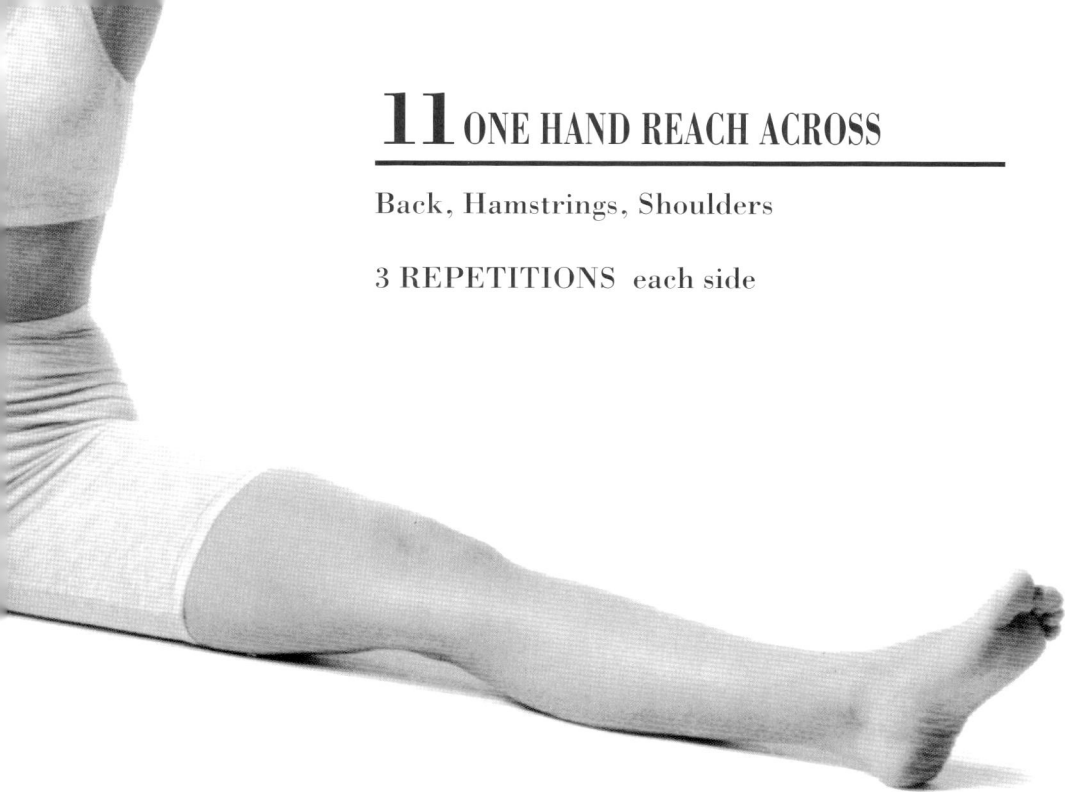

Reach one hand toward or beyond opposite foot with other hand and arm supporting to the side. Lower chest to knee, head erect. Advance arm for additional shoulder stretch. Hold 10 seconds with shallow and relaxed breathing.

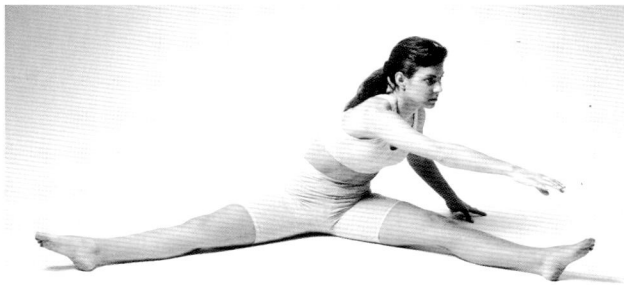

Alternate sides for each repetition. Keep knees straight and both buttocks on floor.

NOTE: It's not how far you reach. It's how well you do it.

For additional calf stretch, actively pull foot up.

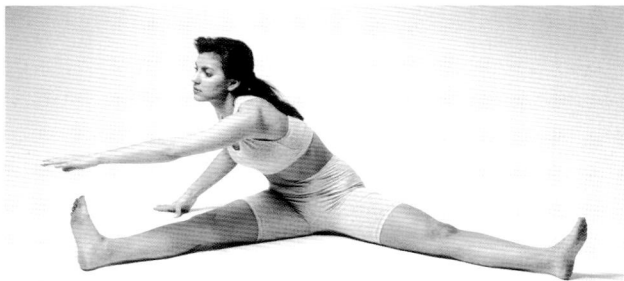

47

# 12 TWO HANDS REACH ACROSS

Back, Hamstrings, Shoulders, Calves

3 REPETITIONS  each side

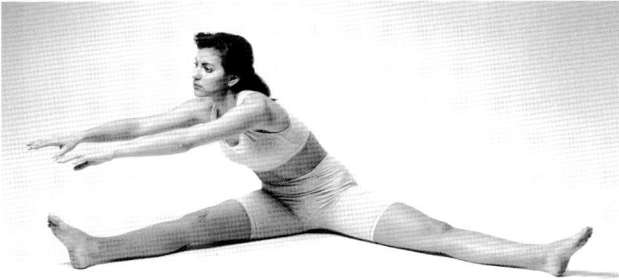

Using the same position as the previous exercise, reach toward or beyond your foot with both hands. Contract your thigh. Head erect. Hold 10 seconds.

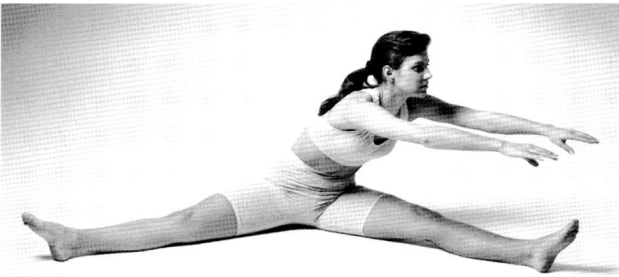

Alternate sides for each repetition. Advance arms for additional stretch between shoulders.

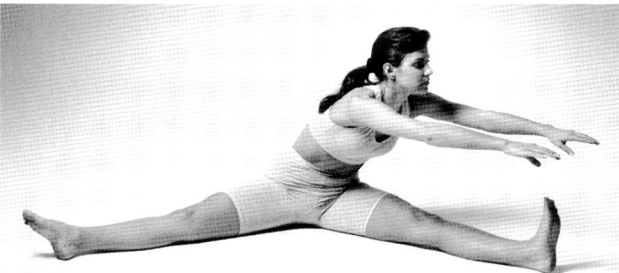

NOTE:  For additional calf stretch, actively pull foot up.

# 13 KNEELING FRONT THIGH AND HIP STRETCH

## 3 REPETITIONS

NOTE: If you have knee problems, skip this exercise. See exercise 21.

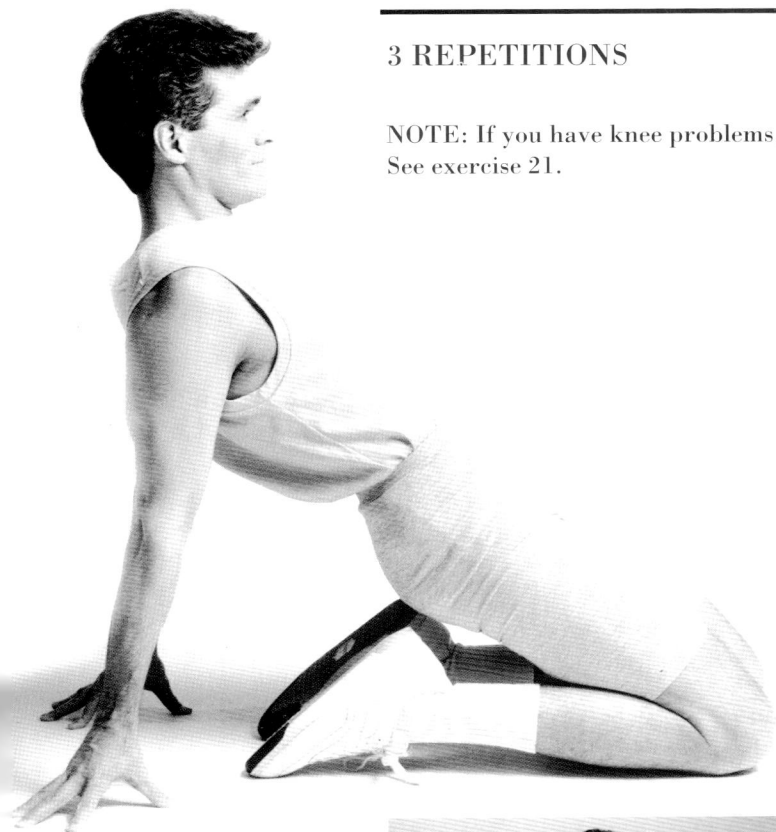

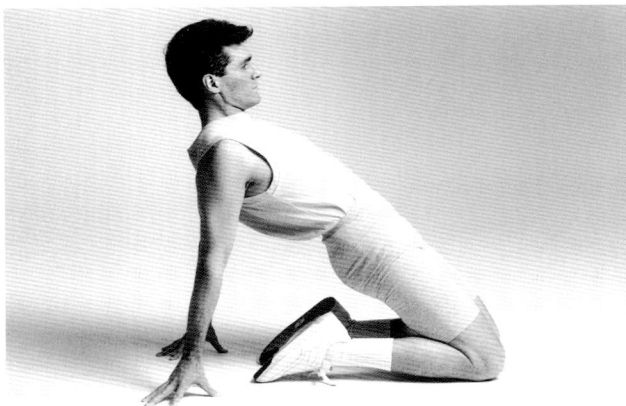

Thrust hips forward. Hold for 10 seconds. Support with hands behind back. Do not sit on heels between repetitions.

# 14 BREATHING - Standing Position

## 3 REPETITIONS

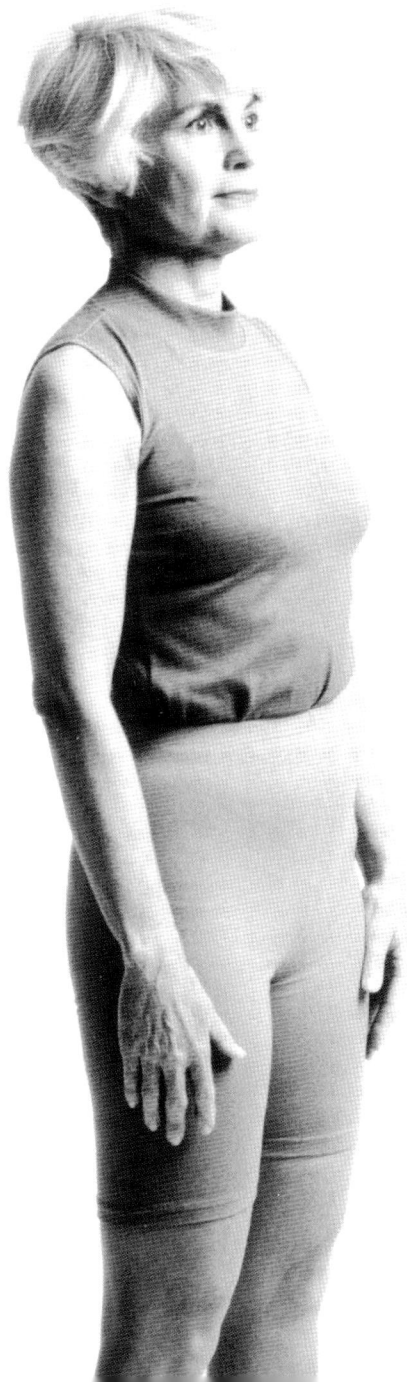

Feet slightly apart, knees slightly bent, breathe abdominally inhaling through nose.

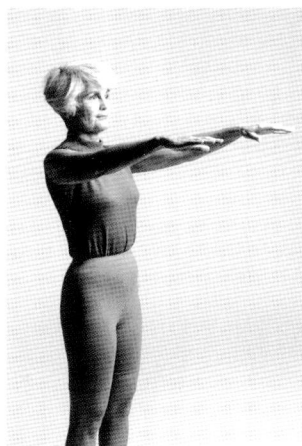

Raise arms forward...

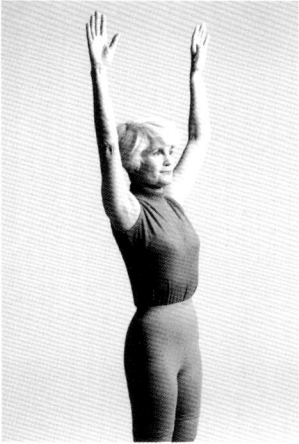

and overhead, pulling air up into chest.

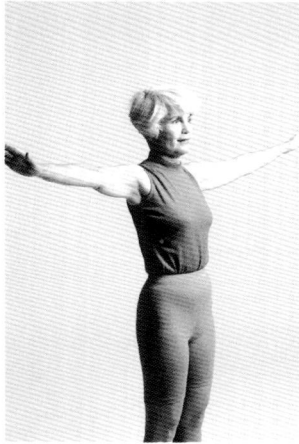

Arc arms down to sides, exhaling through mouth...

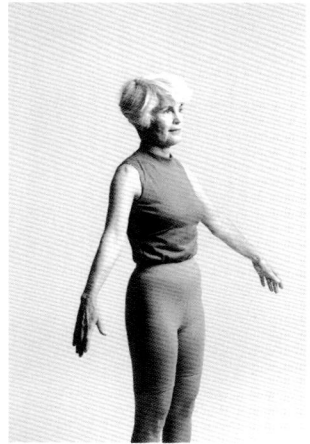

with final forced exhalation.

NOTE: Breathe normally between each repetition.

# 15 CHEST STRETCH

Chest and Shoulders, Posture, Forearm
Flexors, Hands

## 1 REPETITION
each position

Feet slightly
apart, knees
bent, palms
facing forward,
back flat. Reach
back for
10 seconds.

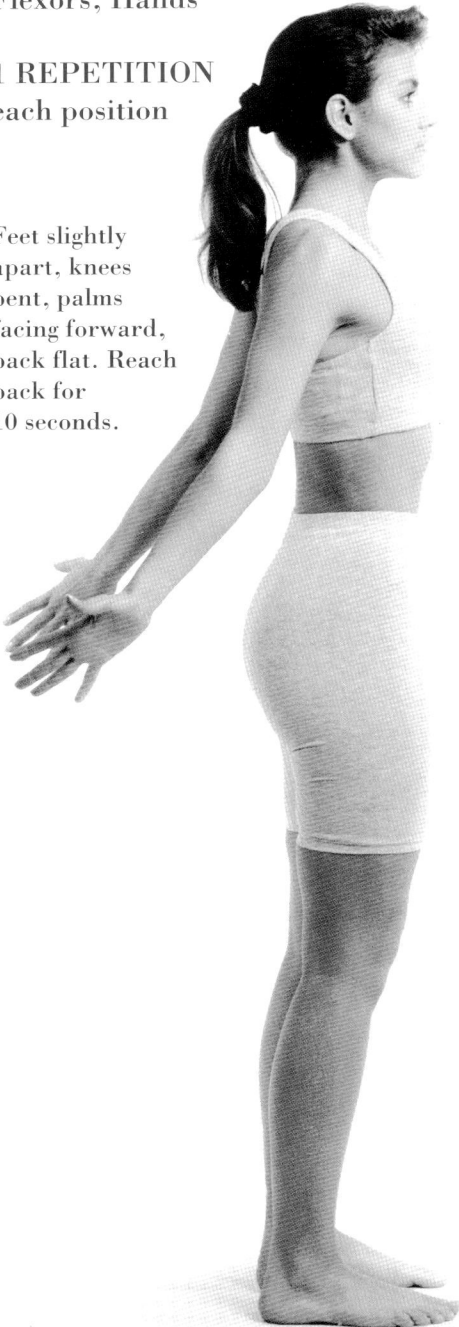

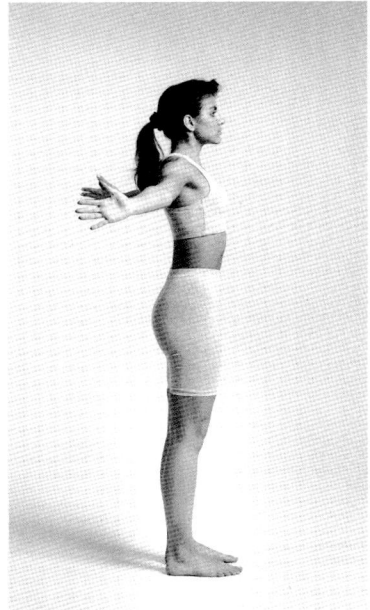

With arms at shoulder height, reach
back for 10 seconds.

NOTE: Extending wrists in each
position will stretch your forearm
flexors.

NOTE: Extending fingers in each
position will stretch your finger
flexors.

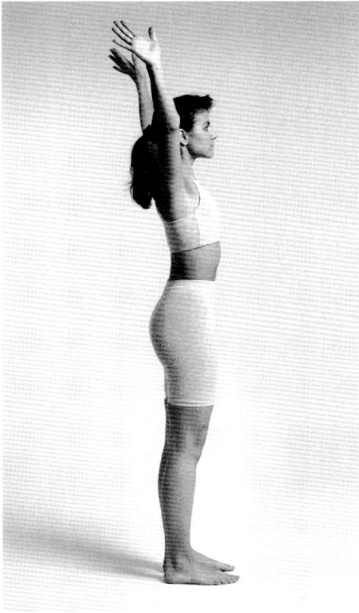

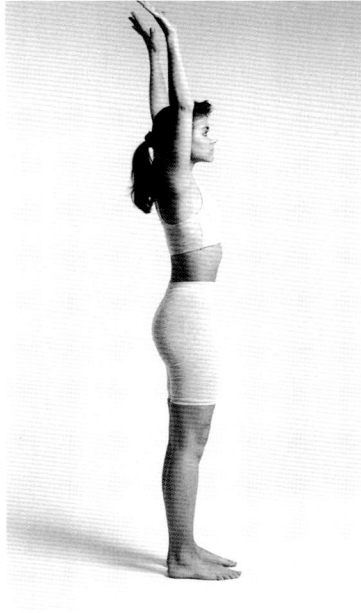

With arms above shoulder height, reach back for 10 seconds.

With arms overhead, reach back for 10 seconds.

NOTE: Breathe slowly in a relaxed manner. The tendency is to breathe too quickly and with too much tension in the chest.

Do not hyperextend your back. The bent knees position will help to prevent this.

# WINDMILLS

If arms are tired, do the following:

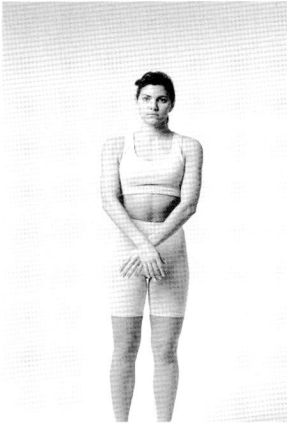

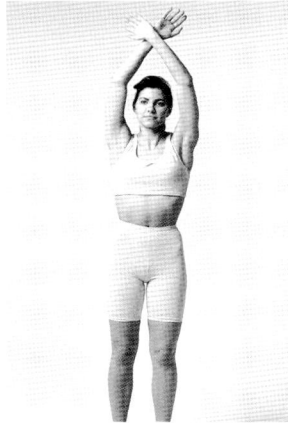

With feet comfortably apart, windmill arms crossing in front of body a few times.

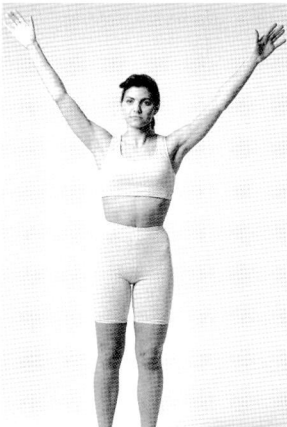

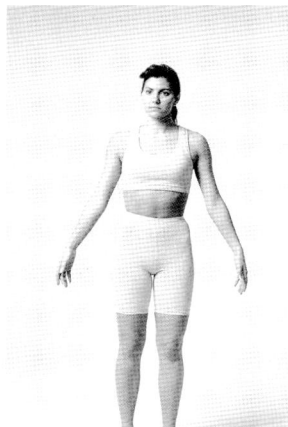

Let arms feel heavy and relaxed. Perform as large circles as possible at moderate speed.

Repeat in opposite direction.

# 16 TENNIS ELBOW

## Forearm Extensors

## 3 REPETITIONS

NOTE: This exercise may be repeated just before going out on the court.

Arms forward, elbows straight. Without making a fist, pull both hands up firmly.

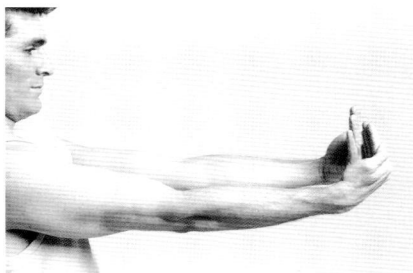

Inwardly rotate both arms slowly.

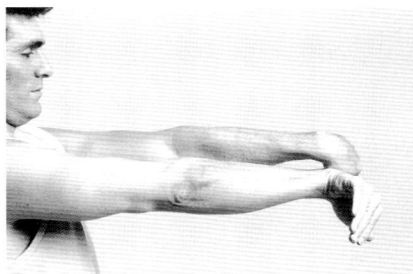

Be sure to keep both elbows straight. Hold 10 seconds.

# 17 NECK EXERCISES

## 5 REPETITIONS in each direction

NOTE: Move smoothly and slowly through the positions without holding for the usual 10 seconds.

With good starting posture (See p. 67), proceed with the following exercises.

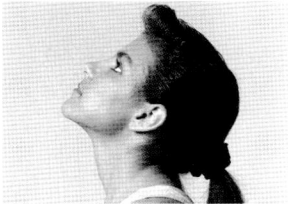

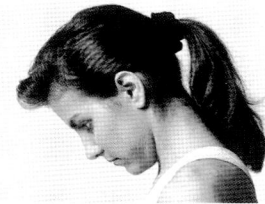

Very slowly tilt head backward and forward through as full range of motion as possible without discomfort.

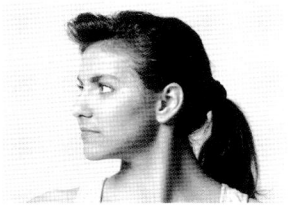

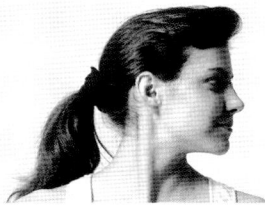

Slowly rotate head to right and left without discomfort. Do not force movement.

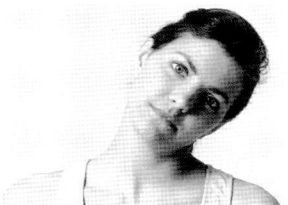

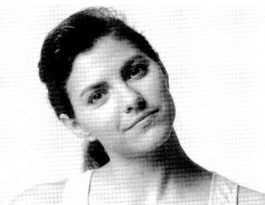

With eyes focused on a fixed point, or preferably looking into a mirror, laterally tilt ear to shoulder. Alternate. Do not allow head to rotate. Do not force movement.

NOTE: Do not perform circular movements. You are attempting to increase mobility in three separate planes of motion, not to test the compound movements of 29 joints of the cervical spine!

# 18 TRUNK ROTATION

Trunk, Shoulders

3 REPETITIONS in each direction

Feet slightly apart. Knees partially bent and low back flat. Do not rotate hips, but...

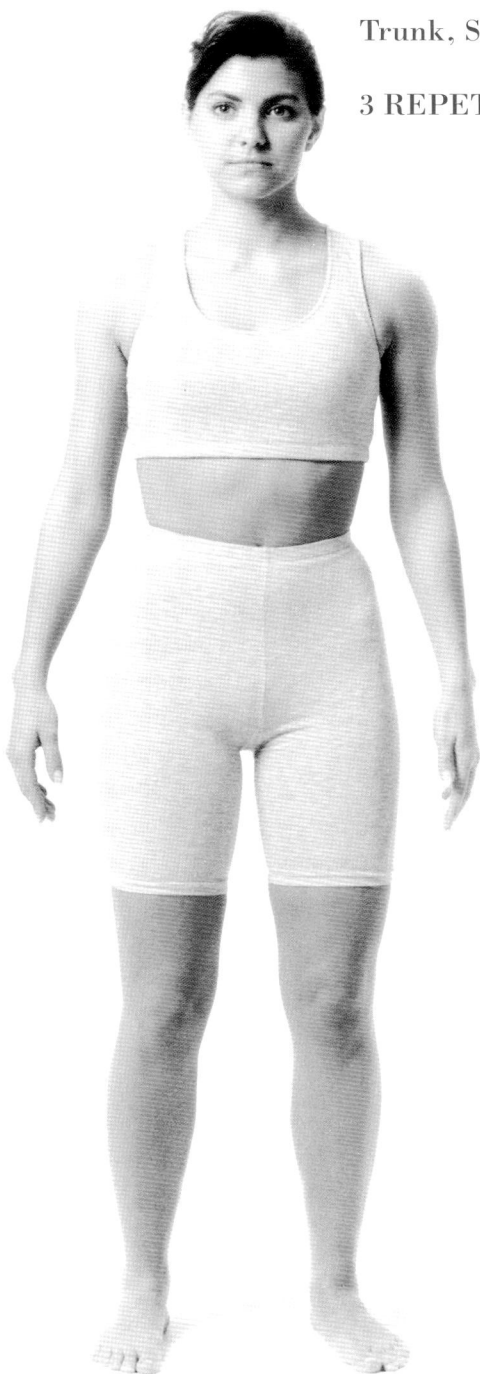

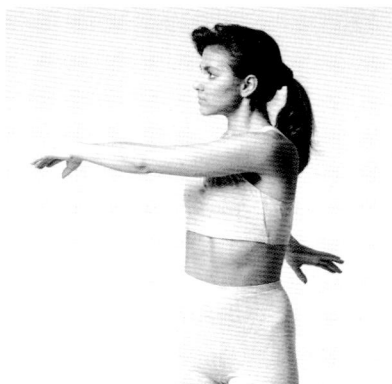

Rotate trunk reaching with one arm in front and the other arm behind you. Hold 10 seconds.

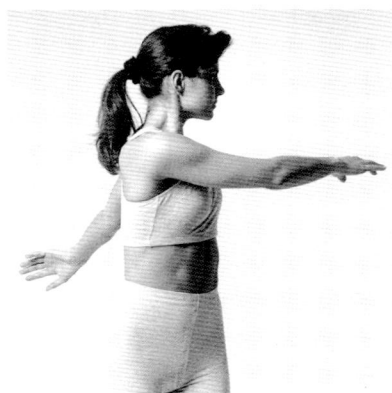

Rotate to opposite side. Hold 10 seconds.

NOTE: Advance arm in front for additional shoulder stretch.

# **19** ONE ARM OVERHEAD REACH

Trunk

3 REPETITIONS each side

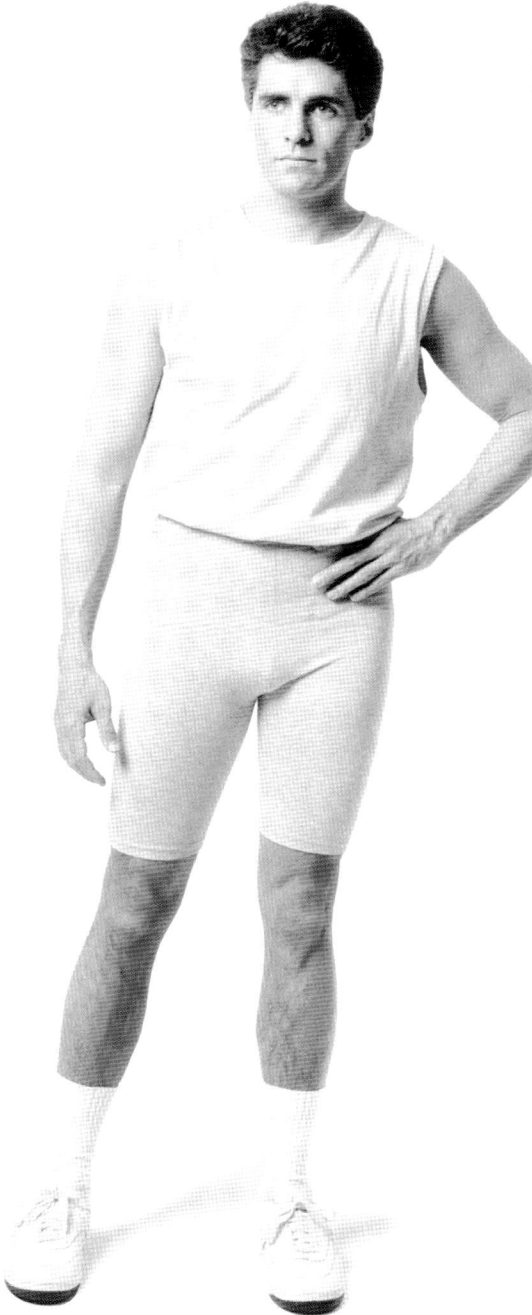

Feet apart, with one hand on hip, drift vertical alignment to that side.

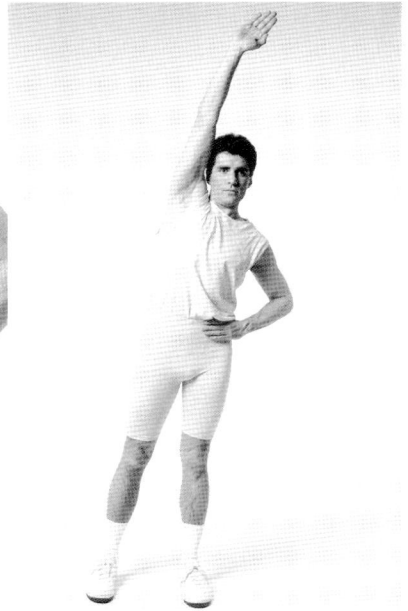

Reach up and over your head toward ceiling. Hold for 10 seconds. Keep elbows back.

NOTE: Drifting and maintaining the vertical line limits distortion of the spine and overstretching of ligaments.

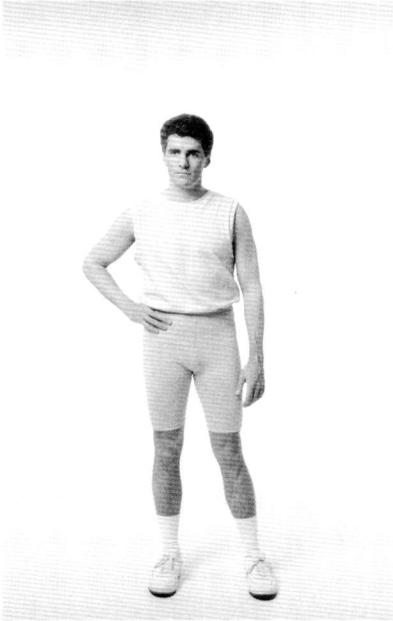

Reverse positions of hands. Drift vertical alignment to other side.

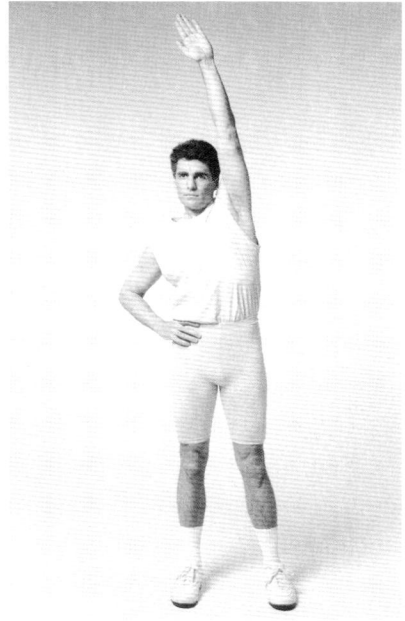

Reach up and over your head toward ceiling. Hold for 10 seconds.

# **20** STARTER'S POSITION

Hamstrings, Hip Flexors, Calves

## 3 REPETITIONS  each leg

NOTE: If you have back problems, or if your
hamstrings are so tight that you can't balance safely,
postpone or skip this exercise.

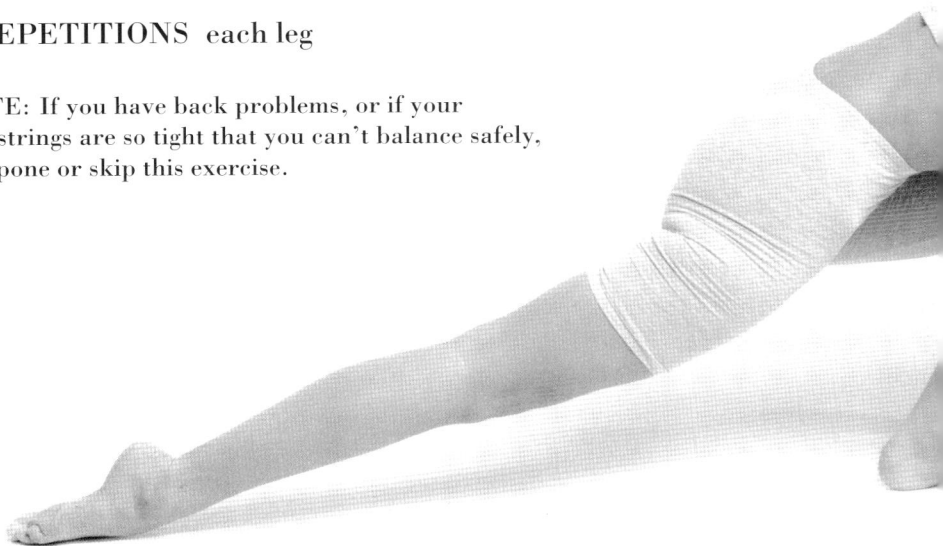

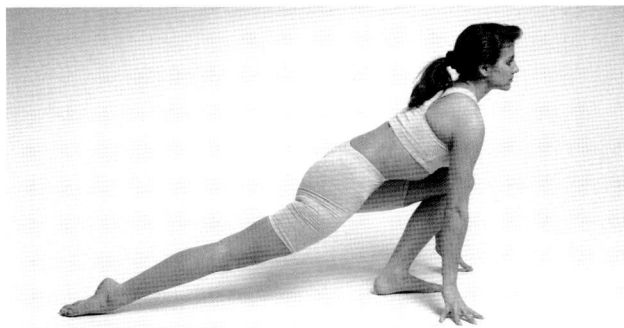

With forward foot flat
on floor and in line with
hands, fully extend rear
leg, lower hips, and
straighten back. Hold for
10 seconds. Keep heel of
forward leg flat on floor.
Pull the bent knee toward
the midline so it does not
rest against your arm.

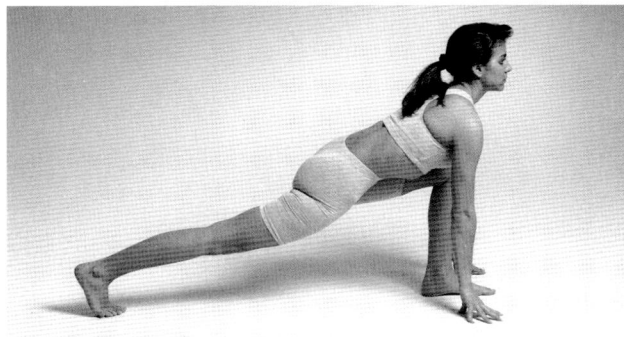

NOTE: If you get muscle
cramps in the front of the
extended lower leg initially,
use this optional position
up on toes.

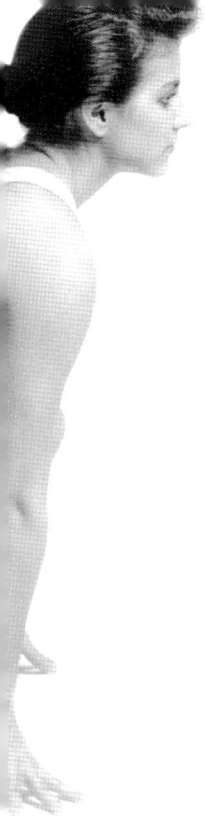

Next, drop to rear knee, fully extend opposite leg between arms. Contract thigh. With head up, lean forward. Hold for 10 seconds. Repeat with other leg.

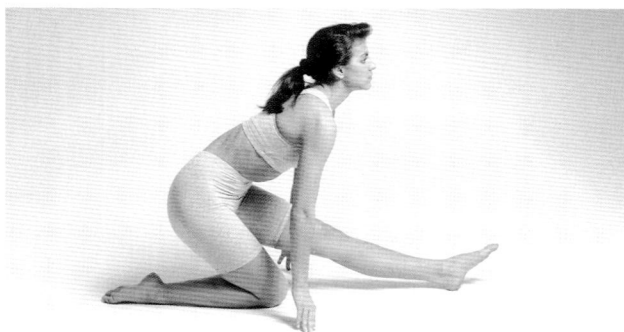

NOTE: For increased calf stretch, you may pull foot up.

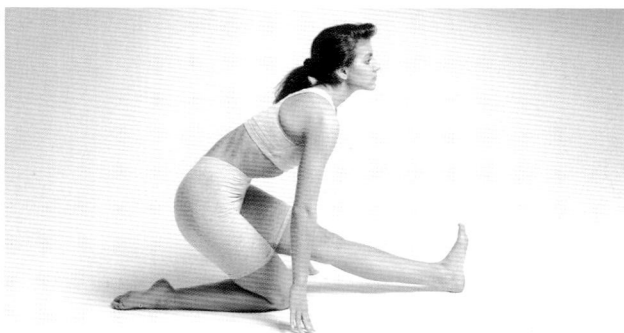

# 21 STANDING FRONT THIGH AND HIP STRETCH

3 REPETITIONS  each leg

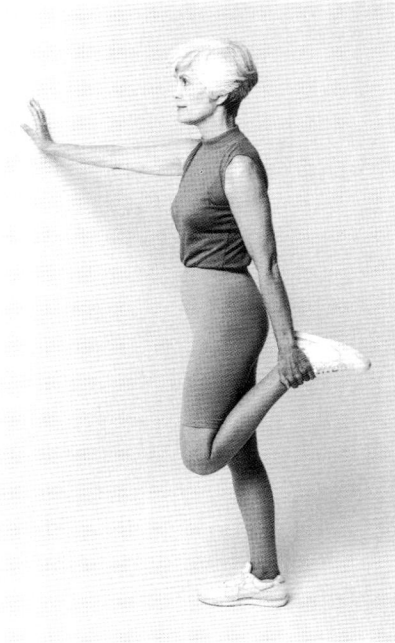

Stand erect with light support. Cradle one leg at the ankle, but do not pull up on it. Keep knees close together.

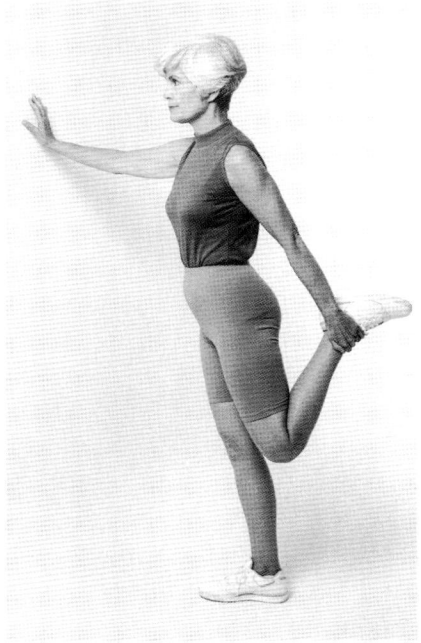

Extend hip. Hold 10 seconds. Repeat with other leg.

# 22 STANDING CALF STRETCH

## Hamstrings, Heel Cords

## 3 REPETITIONS each leg

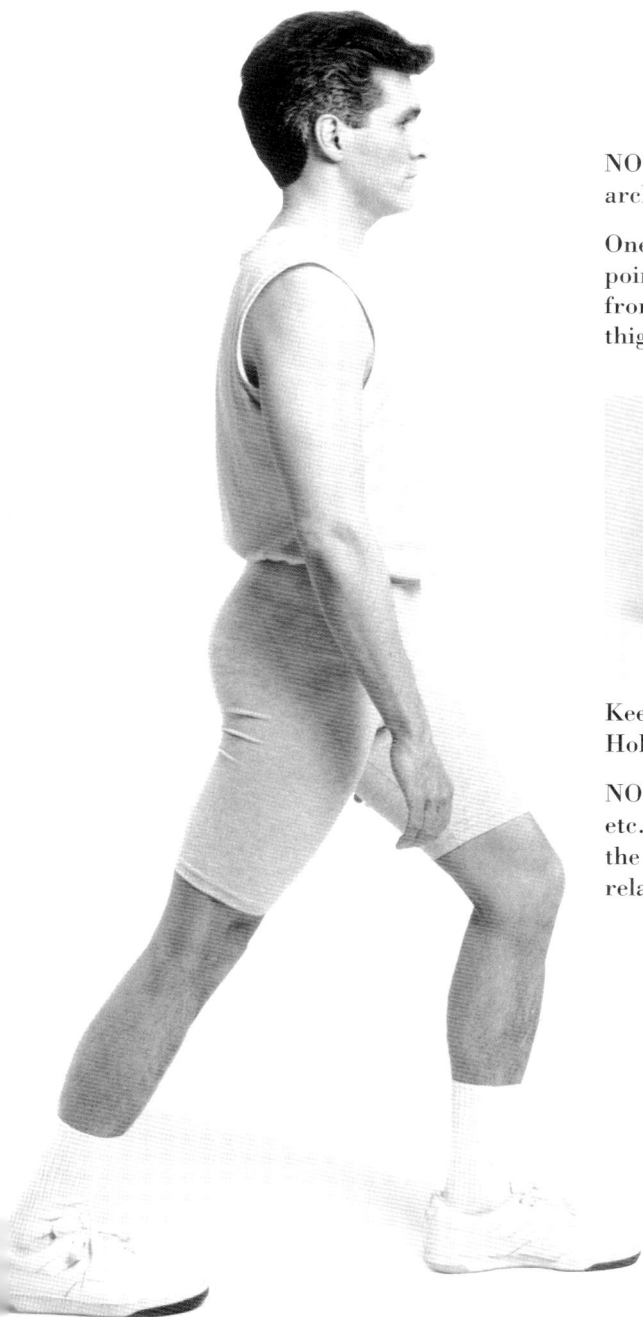

NOTE: Wear shoes which provide arch support.

One foot forward, other foot back, point toes straight ahead. Dip onto front leg while actively contracting thigh muscles of rear leg.

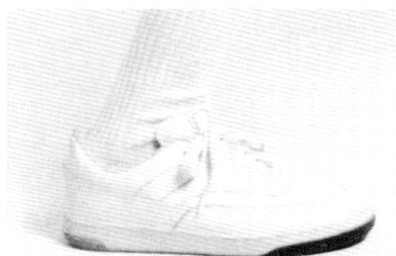

Keep rear heel on floor.
Hold 10 seconds. Change legs.

NOTE: Don't push against a wall, etc., or you will tend to contract the very muscles you want to relax.

# 23 STANDING LATERAL THIGH AND HIP STRETCH

## 3 REPETITIONS
### each side

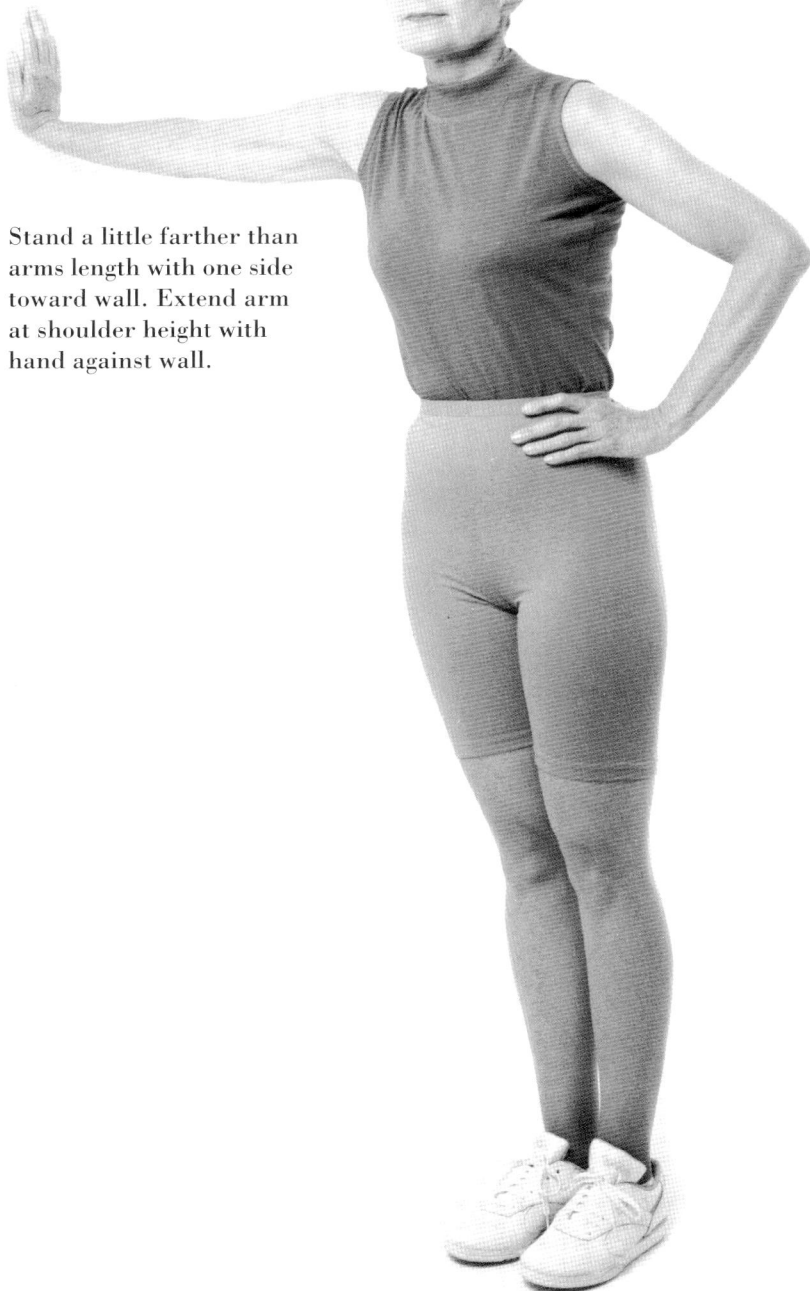

Stand a little farther than arms length with one side toward wall. Extend arm at shoulder height with hand against wall.

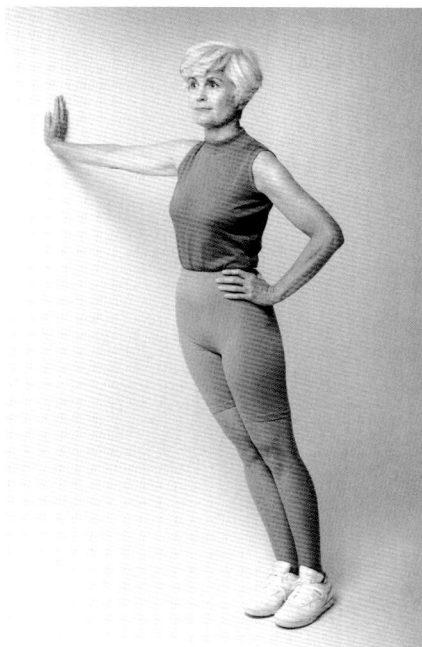

With knees straight, *pull* hip toward wall with upper body vertical and not bending at waist. Hold 10 seconds. Reverse sides.

Congratulations, you have stretched almost every muscle in your body. Undoubtedly you have discovered neglected areas of your body which need this attention. Expect some to respond rapidly and others to show more reluctance to change.

As you become better acquainted with the procedures, you may find that either BY THE NUMBERS (p. 84) or the EXERCISE CHECK LIST (p. 66) will serve as a convenient guide. Refer to the photos and text to maintain the procedures at a precise level of performance.

If your physical condition makes any of the procedures questionable, wisely seek a health professional for their clarification and/or modification.

# EXERCISE CHECK LIST

☐    1. Reaching - ceiling to floor

☐    2. Reaching - supine

☐    3. Breathing - abdominal

☐    4. Breathing - abdomen to chest

☐    5. Pelvic tilt

☐    6. Partial situp

☐    7. Ankle/calf stretch

☐    8. Plough

☐    9. Butterfly

☐   10. Straddle

☐   11. One hand reach across

☐   12. Two hands reach across

☐   13. Kneeling front thigh and hip stretch

☐   14. Breathing - standing position

☐   15. Chest stretch

☐   16. Tennis elbow

☐   17. Neck exercises

☐   18. Trunk rotation

☐   19. One arm overhead reach

☐   20. Starter's position

☐   21. Standing front thigh and hip stretch

☐   22. Standing calf stretch

☐   23. Standing lateral thigh and
        hip stretch

Check ☑ those exercises which you can
do successfully, when you can. The additional
space is for your comments, those of your physical
therapist, or your athletic trainer.

# OTHER TECHNIQUES, DEVICES, AND SUGGESTIONS

Here are some thoughts about...

## POSTURE

With knees bent slightly, comfortably tilt head backward to undo slouch of upper back.

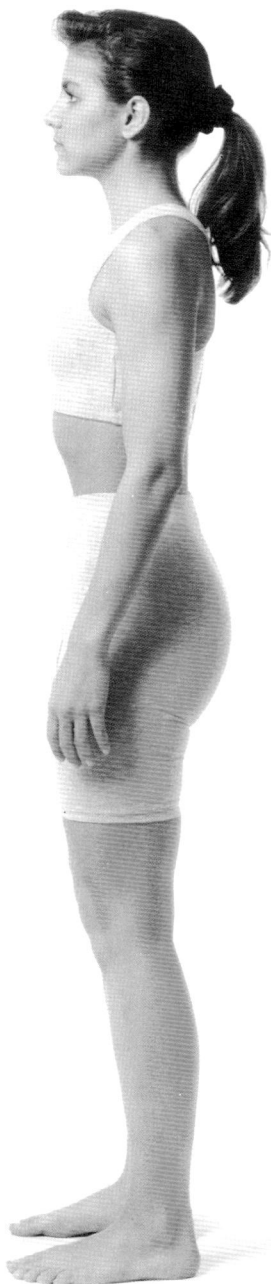

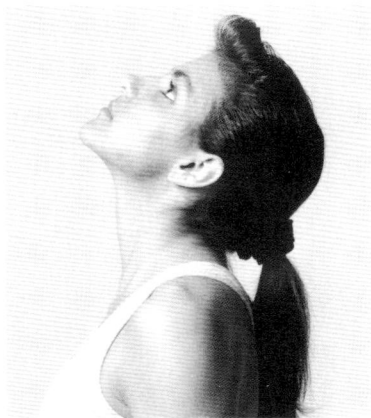

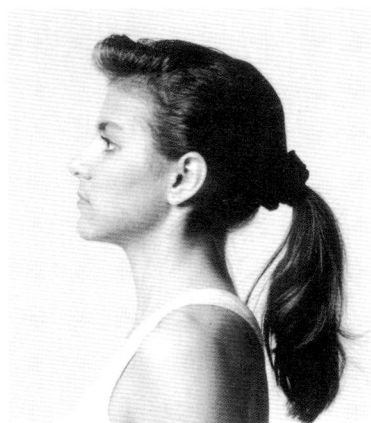

Tilt head forward to level position with chin in. Your neck muscles should not be tight.

## LIFTING OBJECTS

## PROLONGED STANDING

Position yourself with object close to your body. Stabilize your back and bend knees...

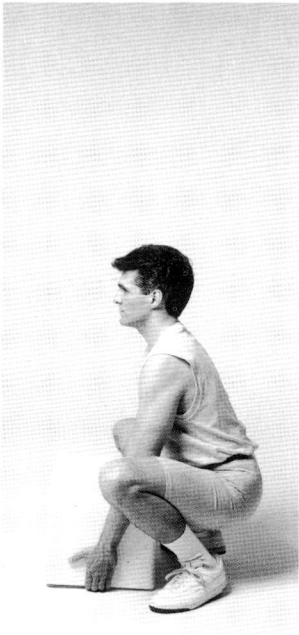

in order to lift with your legs.

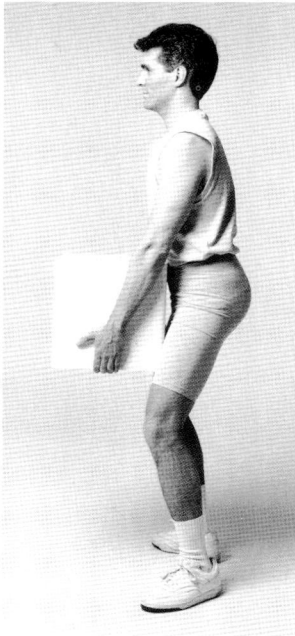

When standing for long periods, elevate one foot on a stool or other support.

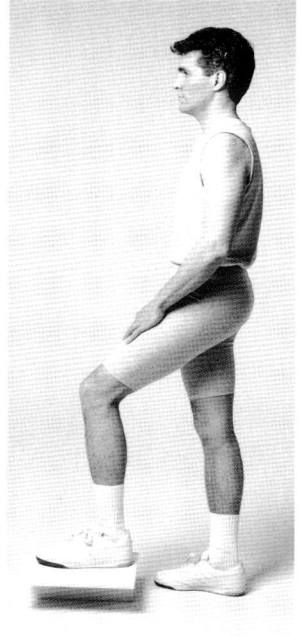

## HAMSTRING AND HEEL CORD STRETCH

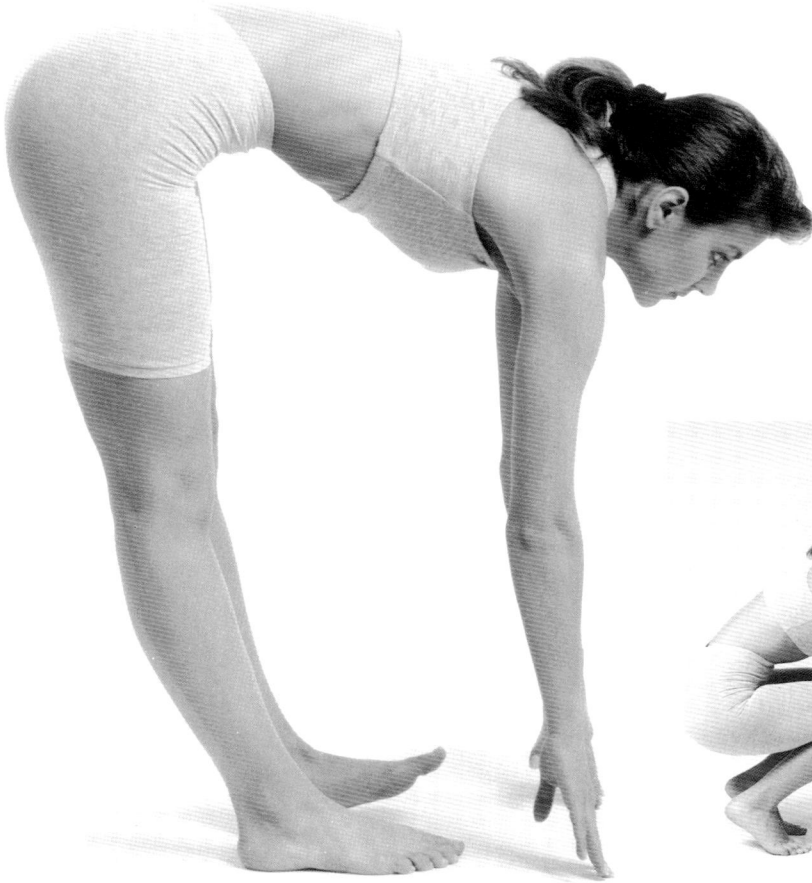

Touch hands to floor, keeping both knees extended. Actively pull toes of one foot upward. Hold 10 seconds. Alternate.

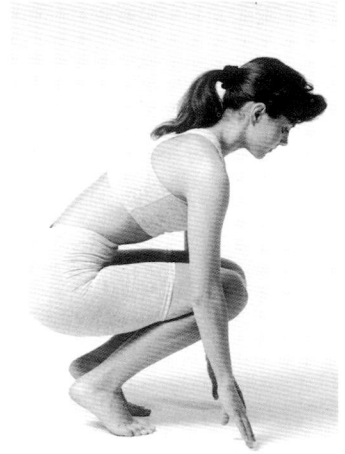

Remember to bend knees before rising to standing position in order to protect back.

## NEGATIVE SITBACKS

### 3 REPETITIONS

With knees bent and feet anchored,
tilt pelvis.

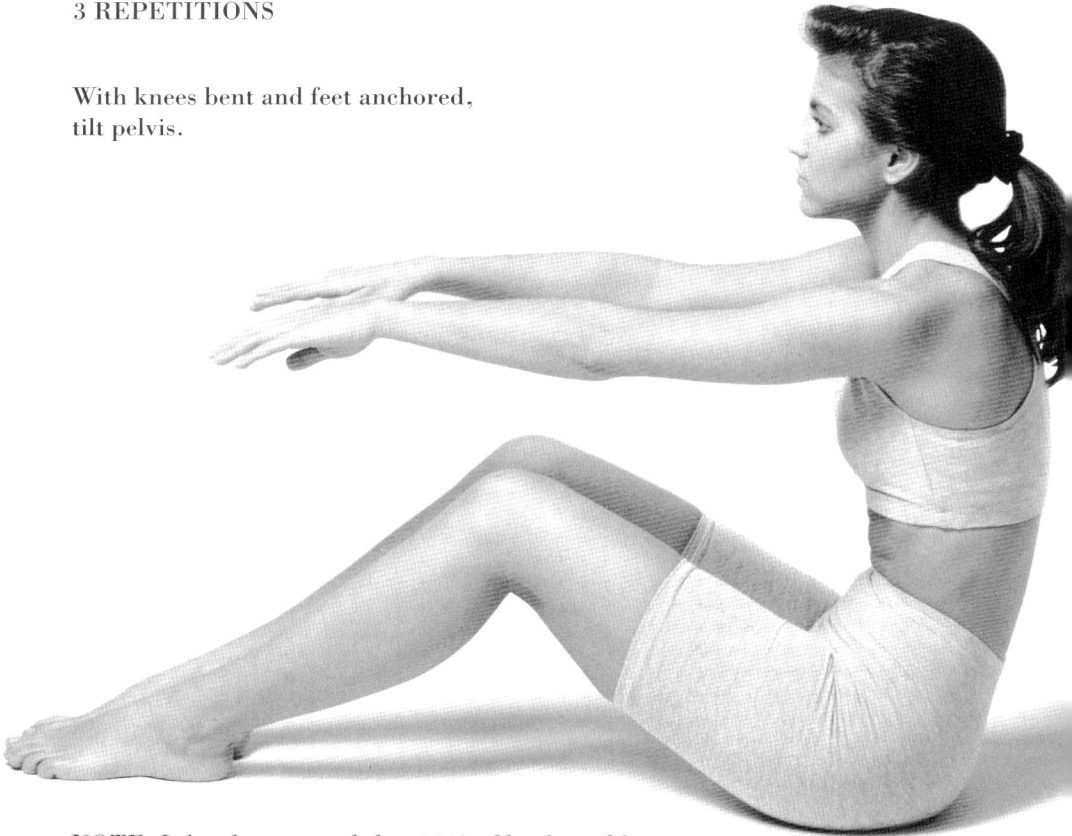

NOTE: It has been stated that 80% of back problems
are a result of muscle imbalances associated with lack
of exercise. Muscular imbalance causes or is the result
of inflexibility. We have had considerable success in
incorporating negative (eccentric) sitbacks into
our programs.

Hands reaching forward, back rounded, chin tucked, descend as slowly as possible.

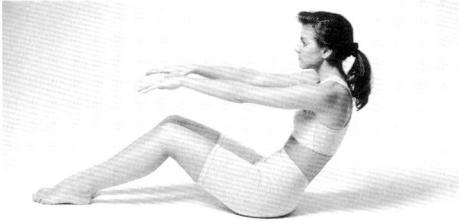

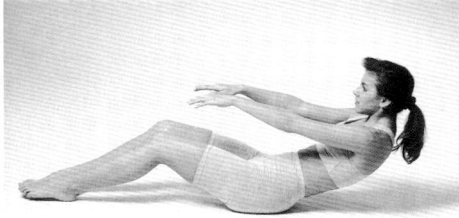

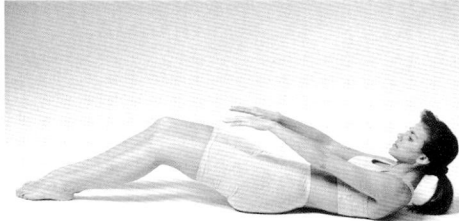

Relax in between sitbacks.

When you are able to achieve negative sitbacks without difficulty, you might want to do them with the variations shown below:

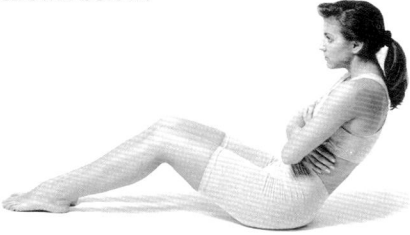

With hands folded across chest.

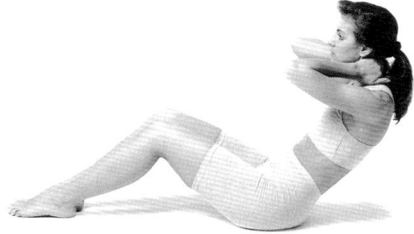

With hands folded behind neck, or by holding weights behind neck.

When strong enough, you might want to try the following:

Maintaining pelvic tilt, hold a partial situp as long as possible up to 60 seconds.

NOTE: If back discomfort is experienced at a particular point, try holding in a position above that point.

## TILT BOARD (scraps of wood to suit)

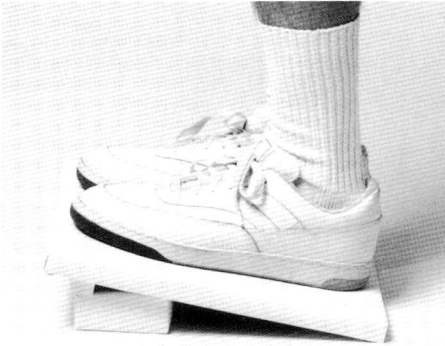

It is desirable to have at least a 10° angle of ankle dorsiflexion, preferably 15°. Under 10°, *prolonged* stretching of the calf muscle is effective, if it is not uncomfortable.

Stand with your back against a wall and your feet located toward the front edge of the sloped board. Occasionally contract your thigh muscles for 10 seconds.

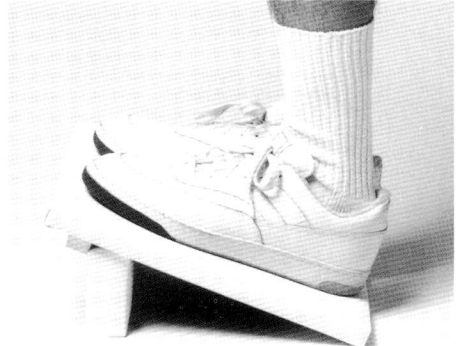

As your flexibility gradually improves, you will find yourself adjusting the angle of stretch (always short of discomfort) by positioning your feet closer to the wall and/or increasing the slope of the board.

These are good times to read or watch TV for up to 15 minutes at a time. Wear shoes to support your arches.

# CONSIDERATIONS

**1. "Active" Stretching** – Voluntary muscle contraction of those muscles which oppose the tight ones. To inhibit stretch reflexes. Relax while stretching. Tension should be noticeable only in the active muscles and the muscles being stretched. Relax in the other areas. Do not hold your breath. This leads to unwanted tension.

**2. Passive Stretching** – Should be avoided. Stretching should be under your complete control, i.e., do not team up with someone for forced stretching.

**3. No Bouncing** – To prevent stretch reflexes.

**4. Slow Stretching** – To permit adaptation of muscles with minimal reflex response.

**5. Repetitions** – 3 times for 10 seconds in most exercise positions.

**6. Daily** – And again before warmup which precedes your activity.

**7. Cooldown** – Stretch again, following your activity, those muscles most subject to tightness as a result of your activity.

**8. Layoffs Following Injury** – You should recognize the need to recondition early, but slowly, those areas which were immobilized while maintaining those which were uninjured.

**9. Pain** – You are stretching too hard, too fast. Skip, at least temporarily, any exercise which produces pain.

**10. Don't Compete** – Your body has its own peculiarities and is not to be compared with anyone else's.

**11. Time** – The complete program takes 26 minutes to do effectively. As you become looser, the time required will be considerably less. You should notice improvement in some areas within a couple of weeks.

**12. When to Stretch**– On some days you may be tighter than others, and you will notice you are tightest upon first arising because body heat from resting metabolism is at a low level. It might take longer, but don't neglect to stretch preceding participation in a morning activity.

**13.  Favorites**– You may repeat stretching exercises throughout the day to relieve tension and to meet the demands of your sport or work activities.

**14. Cramps** – If a muscle goes into spasm (cramps) as a result of your activity, stretch it slowly – preferably by actively contracting the opposite muscle to take advantage of the inhibiting effect of reciprocal innervation. Such occurrences should decrease as your flexibility improves, direct trauma being the exception.


The key philosophy of THE FLEXIBILTY MANUAL is the awareness and maintenance of total body flexibility. When different activities require additional emphasis on the affected areas, you will have learned to recognize the need and be able to apply the necessary techniques.

Mobility is life itself. You cannot survive without it. You cannot perform the simplest of daily activities without it. Your degree of mobility determines the quality of your life. Furthermore, contrary to what you are led to believe, loss of mobility is not a normal process of aging. It is a process of neglect.

*IF YOU CAN'T MOVE,*
*YOU CAN'T IMPROVE.*

# SUMMARY

## THE NEUROPHYSIOLOGICAL BASIS OF "ACTIVE" STRETCHING

Basic neurophysiology indicates that most stretching has been done in the wrong way. This is not new information. It just has been ignored with regard to functional applications. No one should apply static force, bouncing, or rhythmic motions in an attempt to increase flexibility. Force, regardless of how slight, causes the opposite of what one wishes to achieve.

This new method of "active" stretching has evolved from a philosophy of prevention of injuries through total body fitness. Flexibility, providing physical mobility, is the most fundamental component of fitness. One cannot perform or function without it.

"Active" stretching is a method of flexibility training which was developed to eliminate force from stretching procedures. Force, when applied to skeletal muscle, stimulates its sensory receptors, called muscle spindles, to detect (1) change in length of muscle fibers and (2) rate of this change in length. When the receptor area of the muscle spindle is stretched, impulses transmitted by its sensory endings increase in number almost directly in proportion to the degree of stretch and *continue for many minutes*. Also, while the receptor area is sensing the rate of lengthening or shortening, it increases or decreases its impulses accordingly. That is, stretching the muscle spindles increases the rate of firing whereas shortening the muscle spindles by releasing the stretch decreases the rate of firing.

The function of the muscle spindles as described is called the stretch reflex. When a muscle is stretched, excitation of the muscle spindles results in the contraction of the muscle— a normal protective feature but an undesirable response when one is seeking increased extensibility for enhanced mobility and function. The less one stimulates the muscle spindles by eliminating force, the more effectively the stretch reflex is inhibited.

Although it may be desirable, one does not have the ability to voluntarily stimulate a skeletal muscle to relax. Higher nerve centers must be relied upon to *inhibit* muscle contraction. These higher centers are brought into play by Golgi tendon organs. These sensory receptors lie within muscle tendons near their attachment to the muscle fibers. When a muscle fiber contracts, Golgi tendon organs in the opposing, antagonist muscle detect the degree of tension produced. Their signals then are transmitted to higher levels of the nervous system to effect the inhibitory response.

Conceptualized circa 1904 and demonstrated in 1913 by Sir Charles Sherrington, the neuromechanism for this is called reciprocal innervation. Muscles are *allowed* to relax as the result of one's voluntarily contracting the opposing muscle or combinations of muscles. This is the neurophysiological basis of "active" stretching.

Scholars understand this in greater neurological detail. However, it is the application of these principles which results in the effectiveness of the method. The exercise procedures and positions do not appear to be much different from those utilized for static stretching, but the method in its entirety is so different that it dictates some necessary changes in application. For instance, muscle spindles of those muscles one wishes to lengthen should not be stimulated. This necessitates not pulling on any part of one's body or even resting in a position once achieved. Resting one's hands upon the floor or one's body terminates or diminishes the agonist muscle contraction. This reduced muscle contraction in turn terminates or diminishes the inhibition of the opposing, antagonist muscle or muscles one wishes to relax. The "active" stretch will have reverted to static stretching with its undesired neurological responses.

As one applies the various procedures, an awareness of the desired body responses will develop. Once the reasons to eliminate the stretch reflexes are appreciated, the method and indivualized variations of it are within reach of everyone.

There are obvious benefits to "active" stretching. Safety is perhaps the most significant. An individual is not pitting agonist and antagonist muscles against each other, but inhibiting the opposition of one – that muscle for which increased extensibility is desired. The inhibitory responses are virtually instantaneous. Time saved is used to perform a daily "systems check" of the entire body. If tightness or other problem is detected, it can be addressed immediately. The normal process of reciprocal innervation does not require tissue warmth before hand. Therefore, the all-important warmup procedures necessary for safe activity can be performed without interruption or neglect.

When extraneous forces are not imposed, voluntary contraction of an agonist cannot overpower and injure a normal antagonist muscle. So, active procedures are self-limiting. This answers the often-asked question, "How much is enough?" There is no outside force applied by others or through body positioning, which could be beyond the control of the individual. Also, each procedure in the progressive sequence is achieved comfortably.

Why must one stretch daily? Fibrous connective tissue is the single most prevalent tissue in the body and provides structural support in the form of bone, cartilage, tendon, and fascia. The implication of connective tissue and its fibrous protein components in human mobility is significant. One of these, collagen, is estimated to account for as much as 25% of body protein. The *continuous process* of connective tissue replacement, and reorganization of its collagen meshwork into a shortened state, requires daily countermeasures to prevent loss of body mobility. A quick-fix reversal of shortened muscle tissue, quite possibly of long standing and under such constant adverse influences, is not possible.

As mentioned previously, two causes of strain are (1) loss of coordination from fatigue and (2) exceeding the extensibility of muscles and tendons. "Active" stretching addresses the problem of non-contact muscle strains in sports and daily activities. By increasing physical mobility, it undoubtedly has some positive bearing on general conditioning and consequent reduction of other types of injuries also.

# BIBLIOGRAPHY

Granit, Ragnor. CHARLES SCOTT SHERRINGTON: AN APPRAISAL. London, Thomas Nelson & Sons, Ltd., 1966.

Guyton, Arthur C. TEXTBOOK OF MEDICAL PHYSIOLOGY, 8th ed. Philadelphia, W.B. Saunders Co., 1991.

Chapter 54 presents concise review material. The following section headings pertain to the neuromuscular mechanisms most pertinent to "active" stretching:

*The Muscle Receptors – Muscle Spindles and Golgi Tendon Organs – and Their Roles in Muscle Control*

> Receptor function of the muscle spindle

> The muscle stretch reflex (also called myotatic reflex)

> Role of the muscle spindle in voluntary motor activity

> Clinical applications of the stretch reflex

> The Golgi tendon reflex

> Function of the muscle spindles and the Golgi tendon organs in conjunction with motor control from higher levels of the brain

*Reciprocal Inhibition and Reciprocal Innervation*

Sherrington, Charles S. THE INTEGRATIVE ACTION OF THE NERVOUS SYSTEM. New Haven, Yale University Press, 1904 (reprint paperback editions through 1961); New York, Charles Scribner's Sons, 1906.

# ANOTHER USEFUL TECHNIQUE

which has evolved from our flexibility program deals specifically with neck muscle tightness. It is an example of what can develop from further interest in "active" stretching.

Notice from the photographs that, while lying on your back, you position your head so that one hand can stabilize it (1.). Then rest your opposite arm with your hand on chest or abdomen and depress that shoulder by sliding your elbow toward your feet. Neither your neck muscles nor your hand should *pull* your head to the side. You merely take up the slack very gently (avoiding pain and stretch reflex response) so that almost a sensation-free, "active" stretch can be applied for 10 seconds in each position. For different angles of "active" stretch, rest your head on your wrist (2.), then on your fist (3.) as you depress the opposite shoulder. Then rotate your head toward the side you are stretching and depress your shoulder each time you descend from fist (4.), to wrist (5.), to a flat position (6.) in reverse order. Don't clench your teeth. Let your jaw relax.

If you want to stretch both sides, it seems best not to alternate, but to finish one side before going on to the other. Return your head to neutral position very gently (7.). Stay in this neutral position for awhile and enjoy the sensation of relaxation often described as one of coolness. You may repeat the sequence, provided it is done properly each time without discomfort. Then do the opposite side if you choose.

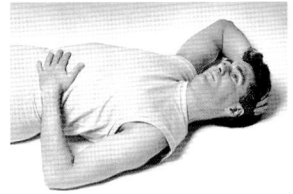

1. Flat, with head tilted looking straight up.

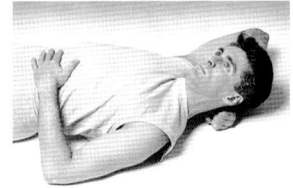

3. Fist, with head tilted looking straight up.

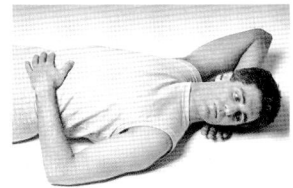

5. Wrist, with head rotated.

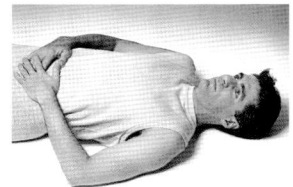

7. Ending Position.

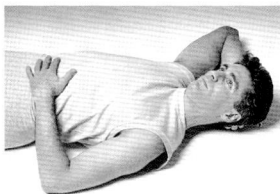

2. Wrist, with head
tilted looking straight up.

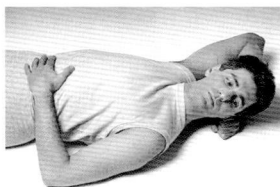

4. Fist, with head
rotated.

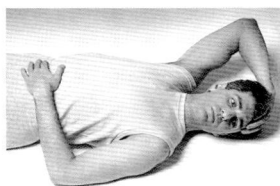

6. Flat, with head
rotated.

The procedure is not effective while standing or sitting because you are not able to relax secondary stabilizing muscles satisfactorily. If you think you must feel the stretch and overdo things, you will have to start all over again and do it much, much more gently. Don't expect miracles. A little over an extended period and on a regular basis produces the best results. At bedtime or even on awakening are particularly good times.

In summary, elevate your head from flat, on your wrist and on your fist, looking in a tilted, straight up position. Then with head comfortably rotated toward the side to be stretched, you descend in reverse order. Be sure the head is supported effortlessly, with no tension in any of the neck muscles, before gently depressing the shoulder for 10 seconds in each position. Remember, no pain or discomfort. This defeats the normal neuromuscular process. Don't be impatient.

NOTE: After some thoughtful practice, you will be able to slide your wrist and rotate your fist under your head while positioning it in a tension-free manner.

# INSTRUCTOR'S GUIDE

## WHAT HOW WHEN WHY

Muscles are stimulated to contract. They are not stimulated to relax. Inhibition occurs at higher levels of the nervous system only to *allow* muscles to relax. "Active" stretching permits instantaneous relaxation of one or a group of muscles while the opposing ones contract. It utilizes this normal function of the body.

With the Sports Kinetics method there is no forced stretching (rhythmic, bouncing, or static) which reflexly tightens the very muscles you are trying to lengthen. The stretch is kept "alive" by reaching beyond one's body and without resting upon or touching anything. Otherwise, the procedure reverts to ordinary static stretching. This also means no teaming up with another individual for forced stretching.

Stretch by reaching slowly to the point of discomfort and ease up. To maintain this state of relaxation, hold for 10 seconds for three repetitions in each exercise position. This allows you to concentrate on which muscles are contracting and which ones are relaxing. Avoid tension in other parts of the body while stretching. Don't hold your breath. Pain indicates you are stretching improperly, too hard, or too fast. Don't compete. Your body has its own peculiarities, not to be compared with those of anyone else.

Recognize the two causes of strains—exceeding the extensibility of muscles and tendons and loss of coordination from fatigue. Avoid these risks by maintaining flexibility and by discontinuing your activities before reaching the point of exhaustion.

The exercises should be done on a daily basis, because connective tissue is being replaced continuously. If it is not stretched, the collagen network within it is reorganized into a shortened state. The end result is loss of function. Daily stretching also serves as a "systems check" for early detection and prevention of problems.

In order to duplicate the success of this program, athletes should perform "active" stretching before warmup. The warmup is so important that it should not be interrupted by or combined with stretching. As part of cooldown, the athlete should repeat the exercises which stretch those muscles showing the greatest tendency toward tightness. Whether you are an athlete or not, on some days you might be tighter than others. It might take longer, but don't neglect to stretch preceding participation in a morning activity.

Layoffs following any injury require early and slow reconditionong of those areas which were immobilized. Don't neglect the uninjured areas. Maintain everything else while undergoing treatment. If a muscle goes into spasm (cramps) as a result of your activity, stretch it slowly by actively contracting the opposing muscle to take advantage of the relaxation effect of reciprocal innervation. Such occurrences should decrease as your flexibility improves, direct trauma being the exception. As your activities change e.g., with seasonal sports so may the stretching emphasis change. It is not desirable just to memorize and apply a different set of stretches for each sport but rather to be able to detect every area which is not suitably flexible. Then stretch those areas more frequently.

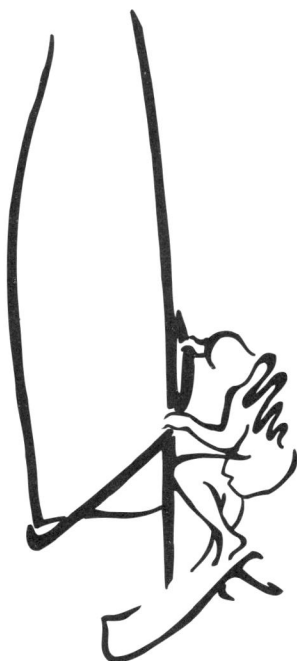

## DON'T PLAY SPORTS TO GET FIT... GET FIT TO PLAY SPORTS.

# BY THE NUMBERS

**To instruct others, or just for your own use, you may use this following format:**

There is a most important thing to keep in mind throughout your flexibility exercises. While you actively contract one or more muscles, the opposing ones relax. This natural inhibiting effect is the result of reciprocal innervation, the normal neuromechanism of your body which allows you to avoid the application of force.

If there are any exercises or their positions which pose any concern, skip or postpone them.

## 1. Reaching - ceiling to floor (p. 32)

● The first exercise is to determine your initial mobility. Arms overhead, elevate your shoulders. Holding this stretch, reach toward the floor. Don't bounce to get there. Knees straight. Before rising, squat fully so your legs bring you to a standing position. This protects your back.

● Again. Arms overhead, elevate your shoulders. Hold the stretch and reach toward the floor. Fingertips touching the floor is considered average. If your fingers touch, try to reach your palms to the floor. Squat fully before rising.

● Once more, elevate your shoulders. Hold the stretch and reach toward the floor. Squat fully before rising or you can put well over 1,000 PSI of pressure on your discs.

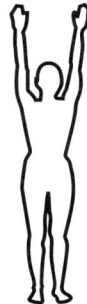

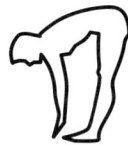

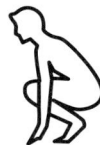

## 2. Reaching - supine (p. 34)

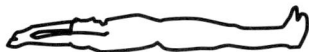

● Lying on your back with arms overhead, elongate and straighten your spine by "walking" your heels away from your fingertips. Release.

## 3. Breathing - abdominal (p. 34)

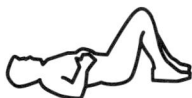

● Lying on your back with knees and hips bent, rest your hands half on your ribs and half on your abdomen. Breathe so that only your abdomen rises on inhalation and descends on exhalation with no motion of the rib cage (3 slow, deep breaths).

## 4. Breathing - abdomen to chest (p. 36)

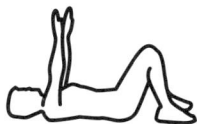

● Same position. Start breathing with your abdomen rising. Continue inhaling up into your chest, raising your arms overhead at the same time. Sweep arms down to your sides while exhaling fully (3 times with restful breathing between).

## 5. Pelvic tilt (p. 38)

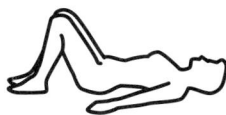

● Same position. To flatten your low back to floor, tilt your pelvis upward by contracting your abdominal muscles only. Don't push down with your feet. Don't hold your breath. Hold 10 seconds. Release.

● Again. Tilt your pelvis to flatten your low back. Hold 10 seconds. Release.

● Once more. Hold 10 seconds. Release and rest.

# 6. Partial situp (p. 39)

● Tilt your pelvis. Then sit up partially. Reach toward or beyond your knees. Don't touch your knees. Hold 10 seconds. If your neck bothers you, cradle it in your hands or skip this exercise. Release.

● Again. Tilt your pelvis. Sit up. Don't try to sit up all the way. Just maintain tension in your abdominal muscles for 10 seconds. Don't hold your breath. Release.

● Once more. Tilt your pelvis. Sit up. Hold 10 seconds. This is a perfect example of reciprocal innervation. While your abdominal muscles are contracting, your opposing back muscles are relaxing. You're also strengthening your abdominals for better muscle balance and prevention of back pain. Release and rest.

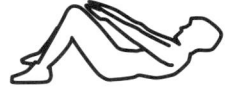

# 7. Ankle/calf stretch (p. 40)

● Still on your back, straighten one leg fully, holding behind your thigh with both hands. Pull your toes down. Turn your ankle in. Turn your ankle out. Point your toes to the ceiling. Pull your toes down once more.

● Change legs. If you can't keep your knee fully straight, lower your leg at the hip until you can. Toes down. Ankle in. Ankle out. Toes up. Toes down.

● Change legs. Toes down. Ankle in. Ankle out. Toes up. Toes down.

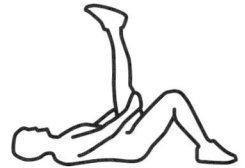

● Change legs. Toes down. Ankle in. Ankle out. Toes up. Toes down.

● Change legs. Toes down. Ankle in. Ankle out. Toes up. Toes down.

● Change legs. Toes down. Ankle in. Ankle out. Toes up. Toes down. Rest.

# 8. Plough (p. 42)

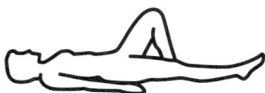

**This can be quite stressful. Do not do it if you have a neck or back problem.**

● One knee bent with the other leg on the floor, slowly raise the straight leg to a 30° angle. Then to a 60° angle. Finally to a 90° angle. Raise other leg to 90°. Slowly roll your legs and hips overhead. Contract abdominals and hip flexors, attempting to touch the floor with your toes with both knees straight. Hold for 10 seconds.

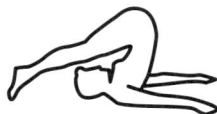

(If your back and legs are too tight, allow your knees to bend. If you have difficulty, support your hips with your hands. If your toes touch the floor readily with knees straight, actively pull your toes toward your head for increased calf muscle stretch.) Bend your leg and descend slowly. The foot of the bent leg should touch the floor before the straight leg descends from 90°.

● Change legs and repeat. Slowly raise the straight leg 30°, 60°, 90°. Raise other leg and roll your legs and hips overhead. Hold 10 seconds. Descend slowly.

● Change Legs. Don't overestimate your ability, but this may be repeated two more times on each leg.

# 9. Butterfly (p. 45)

● Sit up. With the soles of your feet together, straighten your arms and reach forward. Head up. Notice that you don't pull on your ankles or force your knees down with your elbows. Hold 10 seconds. Release.

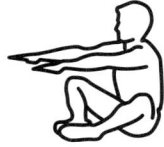

● Reach again. You may feel stretch in the groin area. Actively flare your knees down toward the floor. Hold 10 seconds. Release.

● Reach again. Head up. Don't touch the floor. You want to keep the stretch "alive." Hold 10 seconds. Release and rest.

(In any of the exercises, if you feel discomfort, ease up. Then hold for the 10 seconds)

# 10. Straddle (p. 46)

● Legs apart and straight, reach forward. Head up so you don't slouch. Don't touch the floor. Notice that the sensation of stretch now has moved farther down the inside of the legs. Hold 10 seconds. Release.

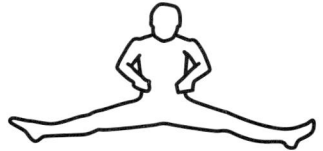

● Reach forward. Keep your knees straight. Hold 10 seconds. Release.

● Reach again. With arms straight, advance your arms a little farther so that you stretch between your shoulder blades. Hold 10 seconds. Release and rest.

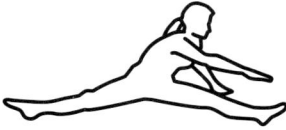

# 11. One hand reach across (p. 47)

● Still in the straddle position, reach one hand toward or beyond the opposite foot. Stabilize with your other hand beside you. Head up. Hold 10 seconds. Release.

● Reach toward the opposite foot. Notice that you do not pull on your foot or show off by touching your head to your knee. Hold 10 seconds. Release.

● Reach toward the opposite foot. Contract your thigh and actively pull your toes up toward you. Hold 10 seconds. Release.

● Other side. Notice that you can stretch more than one set of muscles. Hold 10 seconds. Release.

● Reach toward the opposite side. You are taking up slack in your trunk. Now add some more stretch to your shoulder. Hold 10 seconds. Release.

● Once more. Reach. You also are stretching your hamstrings. So, keep your buttocks flat on the floor. It's not how far you reach, but how far you stretch properly. Hold 10 seconds. Release and rest.

# 12. Two hands reach across (p. 48)

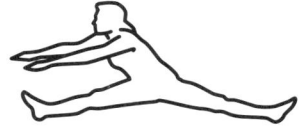

● In the straddle position, reach both hands toward or beyond one foot. Hold 10 seconds. Release.

● Reach toward the opposite foot. Knees straight. Head up. Hold 10 seconds. Release.

● Reach toward the opposite foot. Don't touch it. Hold 10 seconds. Release.

● Now toward the other foot. Remember, you can pull your toes up toward you for added calf stretch. Hold 10 seconds. Release.

● Reach again. Try some additional stretch with both shoulders. Hold 10 seconds. Release.

● Once more. Reach and hold 10 seconds. Release and rest.

# 13. Kneeling front thigh and hip stretch (p. 49)

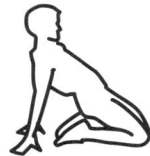

**If you have knee problems do not do this exercise. Exercise 21 is equally satisfactory.**

● Kneel and support yourself with your hands on the floor behind you. Thrust your hips forward. Hold 10 seconds. Release the stretch only slightly so that you do not sit back on your feet.

● Thrust the hips forward. Hold 10 seconds. Release.

● Thrust the hips forward. Hold 10 seconds. Release.

Stand up.

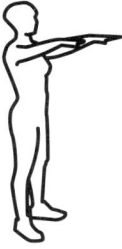

## 14. Breathing - standing (p. 50)

● With knees slightly bent, breathe abdomen-to-chest as in exercise 4 (p. 36). Start with the abdomen rising and continue to inhale up into your chest as you raise your arms overhead. Now sweep your arms down to your sides while exhaling fully. Do this 2 more times with gentle breathing in between.

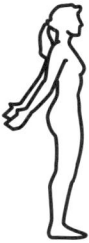

## 15. Chest stretch (p. 52)

● Stand with your knees slightly bent, NO SWAYBACK, arms at your sides, and palms facing forward. Reach back. Hold 10 seconds. Release.

● Arms at shoulder height, reach back. Actively stretch the front of your forearms by extending your wrists. Hold 10 seconds. Release.

● Arms at 3/4 position, reach back, extend your wrists. Now spread your fingers fully. Hold 10 seconds. Release.

● Arms straight overhead, reach back, extend your wrists, spread your fingers. Hold 10 seconds. Release and rest.

(If your arms are tired, a couple of windmills in each direction will help, p. 54.)

# 16. Tennis elbow (p. 55)

● Arms forward, elbows straight, palms up, pull your hands up without making a fist. Rotate arms inwardly. Hold 10 seconds. Release.

● Again. Arms forward, elbows straight, palms up, pull your hands up, and rotate arms inwardly. Hold 10 seconds. Release.

● Once more. Arms forward, elbows straight, palms up, pull your hands up, and rotate arms inwardly. Hold 10 seconds. This exercise should be repeated before going out on the court. Release and rest.

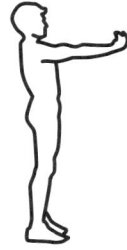

# 17. Neck exercises (p. 56)

**For gentle mobility only.**

● With good starting posture (Refer to page 67), tilt your head slowly forward and backward 5 times. Do not force beyond its end-range of motion.

● Now rotate your head over each shoulder 5 times, slowly and without force.

● Finally, tilt your head gently toward each shoulder 5 times, nose straight ahead, not allowing your head to rotate.

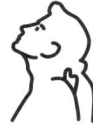

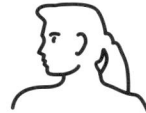

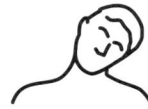

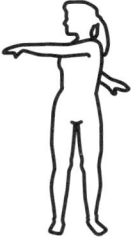

# 18. Trunk rotation (p. 57)

● With knees slightly bent, rotate trunk but not your hips while reaching with one arm in front and the other arm behind your body. Hold 10 seconds. Release.

● Rotate in the opposite direction, taking up slack in your trunk. Add a little more reach with your shoulders as you did in some of the previous exercises. Hold 10 seconds. Release.

● Rotate toward the opposite side. Hold 10 seconds. Release.

● Now toward the opposite side. Be sure to keep your hips straight ahead to avoid twisting your knees. Hold 10 seconds. Release.

● Once again, rotate. Hold 10 seconds. Release.

● Finally, rotate. Hold 10 seconds. Release and rest.

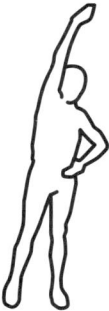

# 19. One arm overhead reach (p. 58)

● With one hand on your hip, drift your body toward that side. With other arm overhead, reach toward the ceiling. Hold 10 seconds. Release.

● Change hands. Drift body weight over the other leg and maintain a vertical line. Reach up and overhead. Hold 10 seconds. Release.

● Change hands. Drift toward the opposite side. Reach up and over. Hold 10 seconds. Release.

93

● Change hands. Drift toward the opposite side. Reach up and over. You should feel the stretch from shoulder to hip. Maintain the vertical line so that you don't distort your spine. Hold 10 seconds. Release.

● Again, change sides and reach up and overhead. Hold 10 seconds. Release.

● Finally, change sides and reach up and overhead. Hold 10 seconds. Release and rest.

## 20. Starters position (p. 60)

**If your hamstring muscles are too tight, you will not be able to balance safely. So, you should skip or at least postpone this position.**

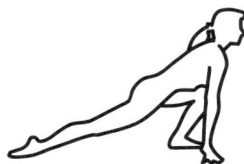

● With both hands on the floor and your forward foot flat and aligned between them, knee not resting against your arm, straighten your other leg fully behind you. Hold 10 seconds. Drop to your rear knee for support.

● Straighten your forward leg fully, balancing on your hands and rear knee. With head erect, lean your trunk forward to take up slack and actively contract your thigh as you pull your foot toward you. Hold 10 seconds. Release. Change legs.

● With the opposite foot forward and your other one back, extend your rear leg fully by actively contracting your thigh muscles. Hold 10 seconds. Drop to your rear knee.

● Straighten your forward leg fully. Lean forward and actively pull your foot toward you. Hold 10 seconds. Release. Change legs.

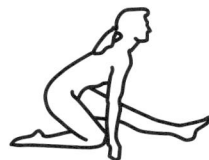

● Place the opposite foot forward. Keep your heel flat. Straighten your rear leg fully behind you. Hold 10 seconds. Drop to your rear knee.

● Fully straighten your forward leg in front of you. Pull your foot up. Hold 10 seconds. Release. Change legs.

● With your opposite foot forward and aligned with your hands, straighten your rear leg fully, head up. Hold 10 seconds. Drop to your rear knee.

● Straighten your forward leg. Maintain active contraction of your thigh muscles. Pull your foot up. Hold 10 seconds. Release. Change legs.

● Move the opposite foot forward and between your hands, heel flat. Also, keep your knee between your elbows. Straighten your rear leg for the stretch in the front of your hip. Hold 10 seconds. Drop to your rear knee.

● Straighten your forward leg, foot up. Hold 10 seconds. Release. Change legs.

● Finally, move the opposite foot forward and between your hands. Straighten your rear leg behind you. Hold 10 seconds. Drop to your rear knee.

● Straighten your forward leg. Actively pull your foot up. Hold 10 seconds. Release.

Stand up.

## 21. Standing front thigh and hip stretch (p. 62)

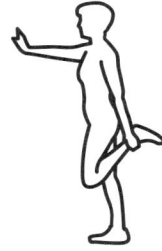

● Supporting yourself while standing on one foot, reach behind you to cradle your other ankle in your hand. Keep your knees close together. DO NOT PULL UP ON YOUR ANKLE. Stand erect and extend your hip behind you. Hold 10 seconds. Release. Change legs.

● Reach behind you. Cradle your ankle and extend your hip. Remember each time to stand erect, keep knees close, and don't pull up on your ankle. Hold 10 seconds. Release. Change legs.

● Cradle your ankle and extend your hip. Hold 10 seconds. Release. Change legs.

● Cradle your other ankle and extend your hip. Hold 10 seconds. Release. Change legs.

● Cradle your ankle. Extend your hip. Hold 10 seconds. Release. Change legs.

● Finally, cradle your ankle. Extend your hip. Hold 10 seconds. Release and rest.

## 22. Standing calf stretch (p. 63)

**Don't lean against anything. That causes contraction of the very muscles you want to stretch and allows the pelvis to tilt.**

● With one leg in front of the other, toes pointing straight ahead, bend the forward knee. At the same time, keep your rear leg straight by actively contracting your thigh muscles. Keep your rear foot flat on the floor. Hold 10 seconds. Change legs.

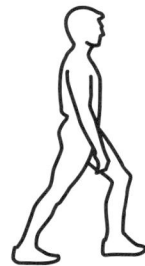

● With the front leg back and rear leg forward, bend the forward leg and actively contract the rear thigh. Hold 10 seconds. Change legs.

● Bend the front leg and contract the rear thigh. Most of the stretch will be felt at the top of the calf. Hold 10 seconds. Change legs.

● Again, bend the front leg and contract the rear thigh. Hold 10 seconds. Change legs.

● Again, bend the front leg and contract the rear thigh. Hold 10 seconds. Change legs.

● Once more. Bend the front leg and contract the rear thigh. Hold 10 seconds. Release and rest.

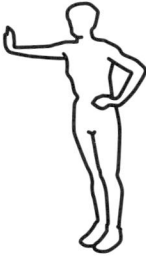

## 23. Standing lateral thigh and hip stretch (p. 64)

**As most runners know, the iliotibial band is a most important structure. We prefer to stretch it in its fully lengthened position.**

● Leaning against a wall, position feet together a little more than straight arm's length from the wall. With upper body erect, *pull* your hip toward the wall. Hold 10 seconds. Change sides.

● With your other arm straight leaning against the wall, *pull* your other hip toward the wall. Hold 10 seconds. Change sides.

● Straight arm against the wall, *pull* your hip toward the wall. You may feel stretch between your hip and knee. Hold 10 seconds. Change sides.

● Other arm against the wall, *pull* your hip toward the wall. Keep upper body erect. Hold 10 seconds. Change sides.

● Again, with your other arm straight against the wall, *pull* your hip in. Change sides.

● Finally, with your other arm straight against the wall, *pull* your hip in. Hold 10 seconds. Release and rest.


This concludes the "active" stretching program. You have stretched almost every muscle in your body, some of the critical ones more than once. Therefore, you should not fret if you could not do all of the exercises. Force has been elimi-nated for safety's sake. So do not defy the limits of your body. They will improve gradually.

# THANK YOU

for coming this far with us. We have tried to explain our system in enough different ways to strike a receptive note with everyone. Some readers will accept and perform the exercises to their benefit without question. Others will analyze it and build upon a growing awareness of their bodies' needs and changes. Some others, we are sorry to say, will overanalyze and confound the simplicity of the method.

THE FLEXIBILITY MANUAL and the video "FLEXIBILITY SETS YOU FREE!" are meant for you, the end-user—perhaps to receive guidance from a specialist if your condition requires it. Although do-it-yourself prevention makes the most sense and remains the goal of the authors, more therapeutic clinical applications certainly will arise (p. 80).

Arguably, everyone is "disabled"—some quite noticeably. Our primary audience is those who don't know it—those who have let their mobility slip away, affecting their performance. We are pleased to have alerted you to the importance of mobility. We welcome you to the growing numbers of athletes and nonathletes of all ages who are benefiting from "active" stretching.

ACKNOWLEDGEMENTS

Design: William J. Milnazik
Illustration: Karen Crandall Peters
Photography: Paul Emma

Special appreciation:
    George S. Holt, BA, MS
    John M. Medeiros, PT, PhD
    Mark E. Reitz, BS, PT
    Lorraine Zowadny, BS

Photo Credits:
    Steve Brown, USA Wrestling
    Betsy Daily School of Performing Arts
    David Demanty, U. of C., Berkeley Gymnastics
    Lyndon Hickerson, Suburban Publications
    Arther Schantz, MD
    David M. Sherman, MEd Ursinus College
    Richard W. Shoulberg, Germantown Academy Aquatic Club
    United States Volleyball Association
    Brian Barber
    Miguel L. Biamon
    Norman D'Agostini, DDS
    Robert Del Vescovo
    Mary Massarella
    Andrew Oberwager
    Danielle Owen
    Howard K. Peters, III MS PhD
    Joanne Priem, BS
    Ellen M. Taylor, RA
    John C. Weidman, Jr.

# SPORTS KINETICS
# PHYSICAL THERAPY INSTRUCTIONAL SERIES
# PRESENTS

## THE FLEXIBILITY MANUAL
2nd Revised Edition

"Active" Stretching explained. Self-instruction format with photographs and text. Group instructor format with running commentary.

**$32.00** per copy
**$4.00** shipping cost

## "FLEXIBILITY SETS YOU FREE!" VIDEO

**$49.95** per copy
**$4.00** shipping cost

## "FLEXIBILITY SETS YOU FREE!" VIDEO
## & THE FLEXIBILITY MANUAL  Combination Package
**$75.00** per set, Includes Shipping

Please Send Me:

_____ Copies (The Flexibility Manual) $32.00 per copy

_____ Copies ("Flexibility Sets You Free!" Video) $49.95 per copy

_____ Combination Packages $75.00 per package

$ _____ Total for Manuals / Videos / Packages

$ _____ Shipping $4.00 per copy
(no shipping charge for Combination Packages)

$ _____ Total Amount Enclosed

Method of Payment: U.S. Funds Only to:

**Sports Kinetics, Inc.**
**725 Hillside Avenue**
**Berwyn, PA 19312-1702**

Please print:

NAME

ADDRESS

CITY

STATE                                          ZIP CODE